DIABETIC FOOT CARE

WALKING IN WELLNESS

DIABETIC FOOT CARE

WALKING IN WELLNESS

The Ultimate Guide to Prevent Infection and Amputation

DR. R RANDAL AARANSON

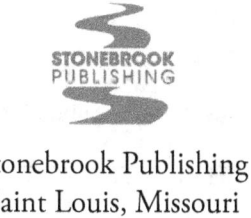

Stonebrook Publishing
Saint Louis, Missouri

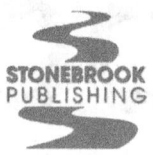

A STONEBROOK PUBLISHING BOOK

Copyright ©2021 Dr. R Randall Aaranson

All rights reserved. Published in the United States by Stonebrook Publishing, a division of Stonebrook Enterprises, LLC, Saint Louis, Missouri. No part of this book may be reproduced, scanned, or distributed in any printed or electronic form without written permission from the author.

Please do not participate in or encourage the piracy of copyrighted materials in violation of the author's rights.

Library of Congress Control Number: 2021907445

Paperback ISBN: 978-1-7370312-0-8
eBook ISBN: 978-1-7370312-1-5

www.stonebrookpublishing.net

PRINTED IN THE UNITED STATES OF AMERICA

DEDICATION

This book is dedicated to the many men and women who treat diabetic feet every day. Their dedication is admirable, and their efforts are appreciated.

CONTENTS

Introduction 1

Chapter 1: What is Diabetes? 3
    What Causes Diabetes? 5
    Insulin: The "Key" to Diabetes 8
    Types Of Diabetes 11
    Symptoms of Uncontrolled Diabetes 15
    See Your Doctor 16

Chapter 2: Effects of Long-Standing Diabetes 21
    Heart 21
    Circulation 22
    Eyes 22
    Kidneys 23
    Nerves 23
    Who's Responsible for My Diabetes? 25

Chapter 3: Skin 27
    The Dermis 28
    The Epidermis 28
    Skin Examination 30
    Dry Skin 32

    Homespun Advice.............................35
    Fissures......................................36

Chapter 4: Corns and Calluses 37

    What Are Corns and Calluses? 39
    Why Do Corns and Calluses Hurt?................40
    Self-Treatment of Corns and Calluses 41
    Home Remedies 43
    Professional Treatment of Corns and Calluses 47
    Looks Like a Corn or Callus but Isn't 53

Chapter 5: Diabetes and Circulation 57

    Evaluating Circulation..........................58
    Pulses 59
    Circulation 66
    Circulation Medications 68

Chapter 6: Neuropathy 75

    Diabetic Peripheral Neuropathy 75
    How Do Nerves Work?.........................76
    Why Does Neuropathy Occur?...................77
    Neuropathy Medications........................78

Chapter 7: Inserts, Arch Supports, Custom Orthotics, and Custom Shoes 81

    The Trifecta of Diabetes 82
    Over-the-Counter (OTC) Inserts 82
    Custom-Made Orthotics........................85
    Custom-Made Shoes...........................89

Chapter 8: Foot Surgery and Diabetes 90
    Common Conditions and Foot Surgery 91
    Charcot Foot. 102

A Final Word. 105

Appendix A: Questions for Your Doctor. 107
    Questions to Ask at Every Visit 107

About the Author 109

INTRODUCTION

Mrs. Poff came to the hospital because something was wrong with her foot. She didn't know what was going on, but her foot smelled funny. One thing led to another, and soon after, her leg was amputated. She had no idea that she should have been taking care of her feet. She had no idea that ignoring her diabetes could lead to losing her leg.

I've been treating diabetic feet for more than thirty years. I've seen how the lack of foot care can lead to devastation. I've seen how the absence of knowledge leads to devastation. I've become an expert witness to the destruction that can occur to the diabetic foot.

This book was written for those who are living with diabetes—and those who love them—to help understand the nature and care of the diabetic foot. Diabetic feet are at risk, but many wonder why they're a special concern. Some think trouble is inevitable.

Understanding the challenges and vulnerability of the diabetic foot leads to an appreciation of the importance of proper foot care. In this book, I share the dynamics at work and help you become more familiar with the difficulties that may occur, so you can be proactive about caring for and keeping your feet in healthy condition. It's not enough to hope that nothing bad happens to your feet. You must be aware and proactive. You are the one who controls the destiny of your feet.

Chapter 1

WHAT IS DIABETES?

The US Centers for Disease Control and Prevention (CDC) estimates that 34.2 million people in the United States have diabetes. This is about 10.5 percent of the population. Most people know someone who has diabetes or knows someone who will get it. The CDC also reports that 21.4 percent of people with diabetes have not been officially diagnosed.[1] This means millions of people are not controlling their disease.

The word *diabetes* is derived from the Greek word *diabainin*, which means siphon. Dia (through) and bainin (to go) means "to go through." This refers to excessive urination, which is one of the hallmark symptoms of uncontrolled diabetes.

Diabetes has probably been around since the beginning of mankind. The oldest known writings about diabetes are from a Greek physician named Aretaeus the Cappadocian (30–60 A.D.), who described the destructive nature of the affliction he called "diabetes." Although he may not have been the first to

---

[1] Centers for Disease Control, "National Diabetes Statistics Report 2020," 2, https://www.cdc.gov/diabetes/ pdfs/data/statistics/national-diabetes-statistics-report.pdf

write about diabetes, his writings are said to be the oldest known to exist. He wrote:

> For fluids do not remain in the body, but use the body only as a channel through which they may flow out. Life lasts only for a time, but not very long. For they urinate with pain and painful is the emaciation. For no essential part of the drink is absorbed by the body while great masses of the flesh are liquefied into urine.[2]

These writings described the most prominent symptoms of uncontrolled diabetes, including extreme weight loss and frequent urination. Uncontrolled diabetes prevents the body from absorbing nutrients from food, and people tragically wither away and die.

Diabetes Mellitus

Uncontrolled diabetes results in the excessive production of urine, which contains high levels of sugar. In 1675, Dr. Thomas Willis of Britain added the term "mellitus," which means "honey sweet."[3] They used to taste urine to see if it was sweet, and ever since, we've called this disease "diabetes mellitus."

Diabetes Insipidus

Diabetes insipidus is worth mentioning because it is a similar-sounding disease that also causes excessive urination. In this

---

[2] *The Extant Works of Aretaeus the Cappadocian*, edited and translated by Francis Adams, printed for the Syndenham Society, London 1856.

[3] Willis, Thomas, *Pharmacetica Rationalis: Sive Diatriba de Medicamentorum Operationibus in Human Corpore*, 1675.

disorder, an abnormal pituitary gland in the brain leads to large quantities of dilute, but not sweet, urine.

When we use the term *diabetes* in this book, we will always refer to diabetes mellitus.

What Causes Diabetes?

Many believe that too much sugar in the bloodstream causes diabetes, but this is simply not true. The high sugar level in the blood is a *result* of the disease, but not the cause. Diabetes is a metabolic condition, which means chemical reactions in the body do not work properly.

Many believe that too much sugar in the bloodstream causes diabetes, but this is simply not true.

Normally, a chemical reaction occurs, which allows sugar to leave the bloodstream and enter the cells through many doors. A specific protein functions as the key to unlocking the doors on the cells. Diabetes occurs when either not enough keys are produced or when damaged keys are produced. The doors remain locked. Sugar can't leave the bloodstream to enter the cells. This is why blood sugar levels are elevated with uncontrolled diabetes.

Glucose: The Diabetic Sugar

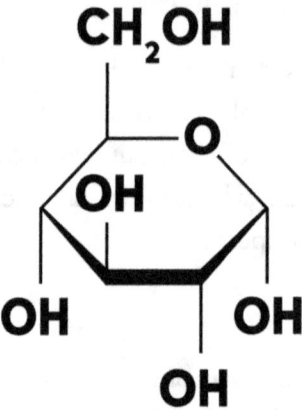

Cells need sugar for energy to function. The cells in the brain allow thought. The cells in the eyes allow vision. The cells in the muscles allow movement. The cells in the stomach digest food. Cells are like engines that need fuel to operate properly. Engines require gasoline, while cells require sugar. Engines sputter when low on gas, just like cells function poorly when low on sugar.

There are many types of sugars. Glucose is the sugar our cells require for energy. Chemically, it's a ring structure composed of carbon, oxygen, and hydrogen. Molecules that contain carbon (carbo-), oxygen, and hydrogen (-hydrate) are called carbohydrates. Glucose is a sugar, which is a carbohydrate. Sugars are "carbs."

Glucose comes from two sources. The first is the most plentiful and comes from the food we eat. The more we eat, the more glucose we put into our bodies. If insulin didn't allow glucose to enter the cells, blood sugar levels would keep rising with each meal.

The second source of glucose comes from the liver, which stores it in multi-glucose packets called *glycogen*. When necessary, glycogen is broken down into individual glucose units and released into the bloodstream.

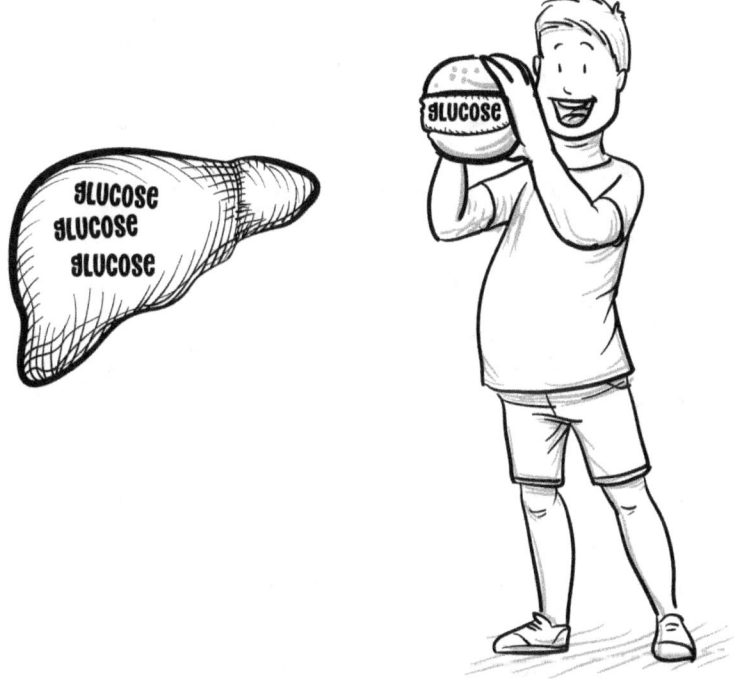

It would be nice if the cells of the body saved only the essential glucose and got rid of the rest. Unfortunately, the survival instinct directs the cells to keep as much glucose as possible. Humans become overweight when excess glucose is converted to fat and then stored in the cells.

Insulin: The "Key" to Diabetes

Insulin

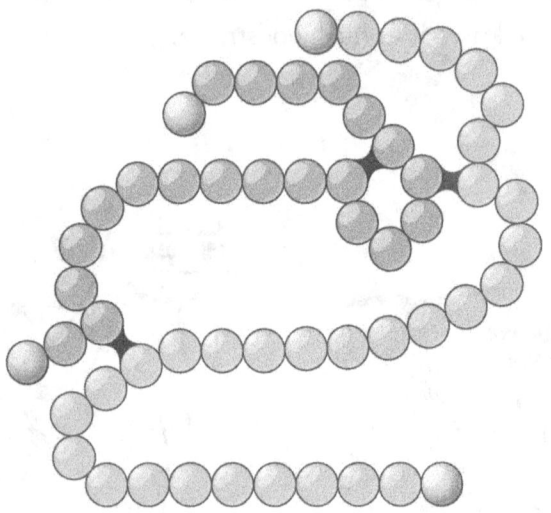

Insulin is the key that unlocks the doors on the cells. It allows glucose to leave the bloodstream and enter the cells. The cells can then use the glucose to sustain life. Life cannot exist without insulin.

Unlike glucose, insulin does not enter the body from the foods we eat, and it is not stored in the body. Insulin is manufactured in the body by the pancreas, an oblong organ located between the stomach and spine.

The Discovery Of Insulin

In 1869, Dr. Paul Wilhelm Heinrich Langerhans discovered insulin-producing clusters of cells in the pancreas. The word insulin comes from the Latin word "insula," which means island, referring to these clusters of cells. In his honor, these cells are called the "islets of Langerhans."[4] The human pancreas has approximately one million insulin-producing islets.

Low glucose levels cause the cells of the body to release protein messengers, which are sent to the pancreas. Once the message is received, insulin is produced and released. Diabetes occurs when the islets of Langerhans in the pancreas produce too little normal insulin and/or abnormal insulin.

Insulin is a protein, which would simply be digested and broken apart if eaten. Therefore, insulin cannot be taken orally. It took fifty-three more years to figure out how to deliver insulin to diabetics. In 1922, two Canadian physicians, Dr. Frederick Banting and Dr. Charles Best, were conducting research on diabetic dogs. The doctors were successful in using an injectable pancreatic extract to treat the dogs. Dr. Banting and Dr. Best, along with professors J.J.R. MacLeod and J.B. Collip, purified the pancreatic extract and were the first to manufacture and test insulin in humans.[5]

---

[4] Langerhans, Paul "Beitrage zur mikroscopischen anatomie der bauchspeichel druse," Inaugural dissertation. Berlin, Germany, 1869.

[5] Banting, F.G.; Best, C.H.; and Macleod, J.J.R., "The Internal Secretion of the Pancreas," *American Journal Physiology*, 59; 479 (1922).

The Pancreas

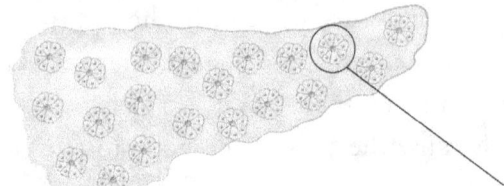

Islet of Langerhans

The human pancreas is a complex organ that produces more than just insulin, but our focus here is on diabetes. Two types of cells that affect glucose levels in different ways are found in the pancreas. The alpha cells produce glucagon, and the beta cells produce insulin.

The alpha cells direct the liver to release glucose into the bloodstream. Remember, glucose is stored in the liver in multi-glucose storage units called glycogen. When cells need glucose, the alpha cells in the pancreas send a protein messenger (called glucagon) to the liver to break down the glycogen and release individual glucose molecules into the bloodstream.

Beta cells, located in the islets of Langerhans, release insulin when glucose levels in the bloodstream rise after eating food and when glucose levels in the cells are low.

The alpha and beta cells work in harmony to balance glucose levels in the bloodstream.

Types Of Diabetes

Oscar went to the doctor for the first time because he had diabetes. He knew the definition of diabetes and the way insulin affected his blood glucose levels. However, he thought there was only one kind of diabetes—you either had it or you didn't. The doctor explained there are different types of diabetes based upon the degree of insulin failure and how the disease worsens as insulin failure increases. The doctor described the three types of diabetes.

Type I Diabetes

Type 1 diabetes has the greatest level of insulin failure, which results in the production of little or no normally functioning insulin. Type 1 diabetes can occur at any age but is historically more common in younger individuals, so it is known as *juvenile diabetes*. Since it requires insulin injections to allow glucose into the cells of the body, it's also known as *insulin-dependent diabetes*. It's as if the insulin-producing beta cells in the pancreas are broken.

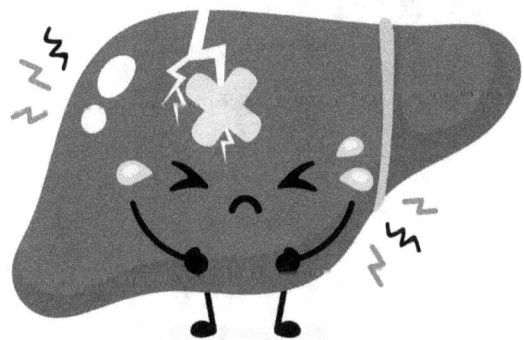

Type 2 Diabetes

Type 2 diabetes has a moderate level of insulin failure, which results in the production of reduced levels of normally functioning and/or damaged insulin. Type 2 beta cells are more effective than Type 1 but still don't produce enough normally functioning insulin for the cells.

Type 2 diabetes can also occur at any age but historically occurs in older individuals, so it is known as *adult-onset diabetes*. Traditionally, Type 2 diabetes doesn't need insulin, so it's also known as *non-insulin-dependent diabetes*. However, many Type 2 diabetics use insulin to control glucose levels. It's as if the insulin-producing beta cells in the pancreas are sick, not broken.

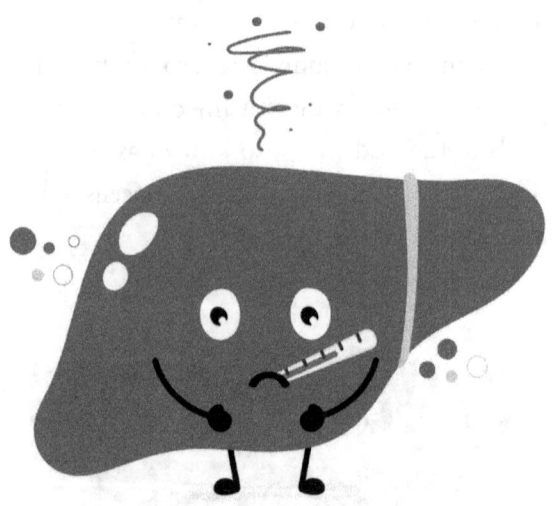

Borderline Diabetes

Borderline diabetes has the lowest level of insulin failure, which occurs when almost enough insulin is produced. Glucose levels are mildly elevated, and this is known as *pre-diabetes*. It's as if the insulin-producing beta cells in the pancreas are tired, not sick or broken.

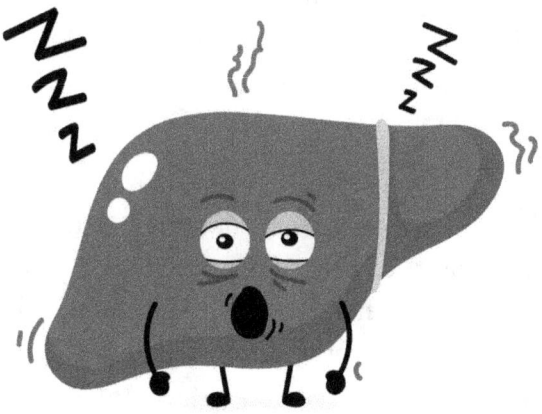

When patients with borderline diabetes come to my office, they're often quick to say they don't have diabetes. Most tell me they don't have to take any medicines and are only expected to watch their diet. They're afraid to admit they actually have pre-diabetes.

Borderline diabetes should be thought of as a warning because it makes people more susceptible to developing full-blown diabetes. The diagnosis must be acknowledged and accepted, not ignored. Pre-diabetics must start taking better care of themselves. Some physicians believe full-blown diabetes may be avoided with an appropriate diet and lots of exercise.

There's no cure for diabetes. The best that can be done is to manage the disease. This should be done sooner rather than later.

There's no cure for diabetes. The best that can be done is to manage the disease. This should be done sooner rather than later.

Diet and Exercise

Poor lifestyle choices often guarantee that pre-diabetes transitions to overt diabetes. An appropriate diet prevents too much glucose from entering the body through the mouth. Exercise helps the body use glucose more efficiently. The increased activity requires additional fuel. As long as the insulin functions well enough, glucose will leave the bloodstream and enter the cells. Proper diet and exercise help prevent a "lazy pancreas" and full-blown diabetes.

Excuses

Foot doctors hear all kinds of nonsense excuses every day. We frequently see overweight patients with borderline diabetes and foot problems. Overweight diabetics tell us (between gulps of extra-large, sugar-filled soda) that they can't exercise because their foot hurts. One patient actually said, "My foot hurts so much that I don't know what I'm putting in my mouth."

Really? Take responsibility for yourself! I try to stop my patients from relying on excuses by explaining what might happen when diabetes is ignored and poorly controlled.

Symptoms of Uncontrolled Diabetes

Uncontrolled diabetes disrupts the body's ability to function properly. This leads to symptoms, which may include fatigue, blurred vision, unexplained weight loss despite constant hunger, dry skin, headache, irritability, high blood pressure, frequent or recurring infections, and slow-healing cuts or bruises.

Some people don't realize that they're suffering from the effects of uncontrolled diabetes when these symptoms are present. Remember, about one-third of all people with diabetes don't know they have it, which is unfortunate because we know uncontrolled diabetes leads to much more than elevated blood glucose levels.

Historically, three symptoms comprise the classic triad of uncontrolled diabetes: frequent urination, persistent thirst, and persistent hunger. The medical terms for these conditions are, respectively, polyuria, polydipsia, and polyphagia.

Polyuria is excessive urination. The kidneys work harder to filter out extra glucose from the bloodstream. Increased kidney function leads to increased urination, which is often one of the first signs of uncontrolled diabetes.

Polydipsia is persistent thirst. People with uncontrolled diabetes become dehydrated from urinating so frequently, which causes a constant thirst that cannot be quenched.

Polyphagia is persistent hunger. Glucose cannot enter the cells. The cells continue to request more energy, and the person stays hungry because the cells aren't getting the glucose they need. Hunger is not satiated.

Historically, three symptoms comprise the classic triad of uncontrolled diabetes: frequent urination, persistent thirst, and persistent hunger.

See Your Doctor

If you have any of the classic symptoms of uncontrolled diabetes, see your family doctor immediately. The earlier you start to control your diabetes, the less likely you are to have major complications. Don't be afraid to go to the doctor. They have seen this before and know what to do. They know you're nervous, have concerns, and think having diabetes is the worst thing that could happen. They know what you're going through and how to alleviate your stress.

The doctor will ask you about your symptoms, listen to your heart and lungs, check your blood pressure, and run some tests. They'll want to know the history of your symptoms: how long you've been feeling this way, how frequently you feel this way, and the severity of your symptoms.

A good history of what you are experiencing helps the doctor perform a proper evaluation and formulate an action plan. My advice is to write down what you're feeling, how often you feel it, and how it interferes with your daily life. For example, how many times do you get out of bed at night to go to the bathroom? How often do your eyes get blurry? How thirsty are you? Have you lost weight despite constantly eating?

After reviewing your symptoms, the doctor will perform a physical exam, part of which is to look at your feet. I can't stress how important it is for the doctor to see your feet every time you visit. In fact, take off your shoes and socks every time you see any kind of doctor—even if they don't ask. One of the best ways to prevent problems is to have every doctor look at your feet at each appointment.

I can't stress how important it is for the doctor to see your feet every time you visit.

Next, the doctor will want to run tests to help clarify the severity of your disease. If the testing shows mild abnormalities, outpatient treatment may be appropriate. However, if the tests show that the chemical abnormalities are out of control, you may be admitted to the hospital. Long-term, uncontrolled diabetes leads to a significantly altered body chemistry. This can lead to coma and life-threatening conditions. You owe it to both yourself—and maybe more importantly to your family—to see a doctor.

The doctor usually orders at least two types of tests. The first will test your urine with a urinalysis. Urine normally contains many compounds the body expels, but glucose should not be one of them. Glucose is said to "spill into the urine" with elevated blood glucose levels.

Urine should also be free of protein. The kidneys filter blood to allow impurities and waste to pass into the urine while keeping protein and other important molecules in the body. Protein in the urine reflects damage to the filtration system, otherwise known as kidney disease, which is more common with long-standing diabetes.

The second test the doctor will order is blood work. Blood is made of two major components: cells and serum. Some cells carry oxygen to the body, while others help fight infection. Serum is the liquid part of blood. Glucose is in both the cells and the serum.

Serum Glucose Levels-The Finger Stick

Serum is obtained when whole blood is spun down in a centrifuge. The cells fall to the bottom of the test tube, leaving the liquid serum on top. The glucose level in the serum reflects a snapshot of the glucose level at the time the blood was obtained, while the glucose level in the cells at the bottom reflects glucose levels over the previous four months.

Depending upon the laboratory that performs the actual evaluation of the blood, normal serum glucose levels fall into the range of 60 to 110 mg%. This means, on average, there is 60 to 110 mg of glucose per deciliter of serum. (A deciliter is one-tenth of a liter.)

Serum glucose levels significantly above the normal range, such as over 200 mg%, usually indicate diabetes.

Serum glucose levels fluctuate throughout the day, week, and month. A serum glucose level taken in the morning will vary from one taken later that day. Serum glucose levels can be in the normal range even with full-blown diabetes. Serum glucose levels are used to screen for diabetes and to monitor the response to treatment. This is what the finger stick measures.

Cellular Glucose Levels

Glucose levels in the cells at the bottom of the test tube are used to monitor glucose control and the response to treatment over time. This gives a better understanding of the long-term control of the disease.

Hemoglobin A1C

Hemoglobin, a protein, is the part of the red blood cell that carries oxygen to the other cells of the body. The hemoglobin A1C (HbA1C) test determines the level of glucose in the cellular portion of blood. More specifically, it measures how much glucose is attached to the hemoglobin protein in the red blood cells. This is more than a random snapshot of glucose control. The HbA1C corresponds to long-term glucose control during the previous four months.

How the HbA1C Test is Determined

Red blood cells are produced each day by the bone marrow and live for about four months. A given sample of blood contains red blood cells of all ages, up to 120 days old.

Every day, glucose attaches to the hemoglobin molecules in the newly formed red blood cells. More glucose attaches when levels are higher and less attach with lower glucose levels. The amount of glucose that attaches differs each day as glucose levels vary from day to day. The HbA1C is the average amount of glucose attached to the hemoglobin molecules during the previous 120-day period. A normal HbA1C reflects good long-term control. An elevated HgA1C reflects higher glucose levels and poor control.

How the HbA1C is Reported

The HbA1C reflects how much glucose attached to the hemoglobin molecule over the previous 120 days relative to how much could attach. Normally, only 3% to 6% attach to the hemoglobulin molecule. Thus, a normal HbA1C is reported as 3–6%. An HbA1C level above 6% reveals poor glucose control over the previous four months.

Daily variations affect the HbA1C to a very mild degree. One good or bad day comprises only $1/120^{th}$, or 0.0083%, of the 120-day HbA1c. Normal HgA1C levels are the goal with diabetes and can be achieved with diet, exercise, experience, and motivation.

HbA1C levels above 6% reveal the patient is not following treatment protocols or they are not on the correct type or amount of medicine. More often than not, the patient is not taking ownership of the disease. Patients must realize that this poor behavior has a negative effect on their body.

According to the American Diabetes Association's website www.diabetes.org, pre-diabetes is defined as a fasting serum glucose level greater than 100 mg% but less than 125 mg% or an HbA1C between 5.7% and 6.5%.

Chapter 2

EFFECTS OF LONG-STANDING DIABETES

The problem with long-standing diabetes is the gradually reducing function of multiple organs in the body. This occurs from damage to the small blood vessels that supply blood to the organs. The altered micro-circulation affects the heart, eyes, kidneys, nerves, brain, skin, and feet.

Heart

Diabetes damages the heart by reducing blood flow to the cells of the heart muscle. This results in a weakened heart. When the heart is weak, it loses the ability to pump blood to the rest of the body properly. The heart tries to work harder, leading to elevated blood pressure, or hypertension. Reduced or blocked blood flow leads to the death of the heart cells. This is called a myocardial infarction (MI), or heart attack. Most have chest pain, but diabetics with neuropathy don't feel chest pain. This is called a silent MI. Because of how diabetes affects the heart, high blood pressure and heart attack are more common with diabetes.

Circulation

Most of the damage diabetes creates can be attributed to impaired circulation. Circulation can be divided into two groups: the small capillaries within the organs of the body, and the large arteries, which act as pipes to transport blood to various parts of the body. Organ function reduces as the small capillaries become clogged, while blood flow is reduced to entire parts of the body by blockage in the arteries. The eyes, kidneys, and heart—as well as the legs and feet—seem to be most affected.

Most of the damage diabetes creates can be attributed to impaired circulation.

Reduced circulation to the lower extremities is part of the normal aging process. Diabetes causes the circulation to deteriorate more rapidly and at an earlier age.

Intermittent claudication is cramping in the calves, which may be the first sign of reduced circulation to the lower extremities. *Gangrene* is tissue death caused by complete loss of circulation. It commonly affects toes but may also affect fingers or other vital organs.

Eyes

Diabetes damages the capillaries and nerves of the eye leading to diabetic retinopathy, cataracts, and glaucoma. Vision is gradually impaired, thus most people are unaware of the subtle changes over time. Periodic eye exams are important in order to detect damage and allow earlier intervention. A simple eye exam is sometimes the first test to reveal diabetes.

Kidneys

The kidneys are a collection of small capillaries that filter the blood to remove impurities. Waste is excreted in the urine, while important proteins and nutrients are kept in the body. Kidney disease occurs when the filtration process fails due to capillary damage. Protein and other important nutrients leak into the urine and exit the body.

End-stage kidney disease (ESKD) occurs when the kidneys lose all function, and none of the waste can be removed from the body. This toxic buildup quickly becomes lethal. At this point, only dialysis can filter out the impurities from the body to keep one alive.

Nerves

Nerve damage caused by diabetes is called *peripheral neuropathy*. Diabetes causes nerve damage in multiple ways. The first is when the capillaries that feed blood to the nerves become compromised. Nerves, like all other organs, need blood to survive and function properly. Nerves are physically damaged with elevated glucose levels. The structure and function are altered when glucose deposits into the outer covering of the nerve.

Damage also occurs with the deterioration of the nerve's outer covering. Nerves are structurally and functionally similar to electric wires. Wires conduct electrical impulses down a central metal filament surrounded by rubber or plastic insulation. Nerves also have a central filament, the *axon*, which is insulated by surrounding cells called *myelin*. The axon allows electrical impulses to travel down the nerve, like the central metal filament of a wire. The myelin cells surround and insulate the axon, like rubber or plastic cover a wire.

Damage to the myelin cells is similar to damage of the rubber or plastic around a wire. If you were to strip off some of the rubber or plastic around a wire, the wire wouldn't work properly. The electrical impulse running down the metal filament would be inconsistent and abnormal. The lights would flicker. Damage to the surrounding myelin layer creates the same short circuit. The nerve can't function properly. Instead of flickering lights, the short circuit creates symptoms such as tingling, numbness, burning, hot and/or cold feeling, and the decreased ability to feel pain. This condition is known as *diabetic peripheral neuropathy*.

Diabetes causes nerve damage in multiple ways.

People with diabetes often have many concerns about their feet. Most have heard about infection, gangrene, and amputation. Some think neuropathy leads to amputation. Not so! It's the loss of circulation and/or infection that leads to amputation. *Medical News Today* reports that approximately two out of 1,000 diabetic women and approximately six out of 1,000 diabetic men will experience an amputation at some point in their life, primarily due to poor circulation and infection, but not neuropathy.

> *Some think neuropathy leads to amputation.*
> *Not so! It's the loss of circulation and/or infection*
> *that leads to amputation.*

Who's Responsible for My Diabetes?

Despite the best of care, damage sometimes continues to progress. However, much of the deterioration is preventable. That's right, *preventable*. In my experience of over three decades of treating patients with diabetes, the lack of care and ownership of the disease is why most patients have significant problems. You are mistaken if you think that controlling your diabetes isn't important.

If you only get one point out of this book, you must realize that diabetes is real, and you are mostly in control of its progression. Whether or not you develop complications from diabetes is more likely than not up to you.

Your doctor, your spouse, and your children don't control your daily decisions. *You* decide what goes in your mouth. *You* decide to sit on the couch and eat ice cream every night. *You* choose not to exercise.

> *If you only get one point out of this book, you must realize*
> *that diabetes is real, and you are mostly in control*
> *of its progression.*

Get off the couch! At least walk a little bit before you tell yourself that you can't make the right food choice or before you make up some lame excuse. The next day, walk even farther, and the next time even farther than that. Achieve some type of athletic goal every day. I'm not talking about playing ice hockey for an hour; I'm talking about walking a little each day and increasing your distance over time. Exercise improves circulation and helps with glucose control. It can help prevent the disease from getting worse.

Aunt Bobbie mostly watched television and ate cookies at night. She washed the cookies down with bottles of sugary soda. She tried to ignore her blurry vision and fatigue. At her yearly physical, the doctor noted she had gained forty pounds since her last visit. Sure enough, a blood test revealed a glucose level of 150 mg%. She was diagnosed with pre-diabetes.

Aunt Bobbie decided to do something about her condition. She walked around the block a few times every day. She stopped eating cookies and drinking sugary soda every night. She ate healthy foods and drank plenty of water.

The doctor was so pleased to see Aunt Bobbie at her next visit. She lost the forty pounds and had a glucose level of 98 mg%. More importantly, she changed the direction of her diabetes and life. She couldn't wait to spend time with her grandchildren at their next party.

Chapter 3

SKIN

What is the largest organ of the body? Is it the heart or brain? Could it be the lungs? Actually, skin is the largest organ of the body. Skin wraps us in a protective coat, which helps keep in the good stuff and keep out the bad. Taking care of the skin is critical to maintaining good health. Yet, many take it for granted until a problem develops.

Structurally, the skin is composed of two distinct layers: the inner skin, or the *dermis*, and the outer skin, or the *epidermis*.

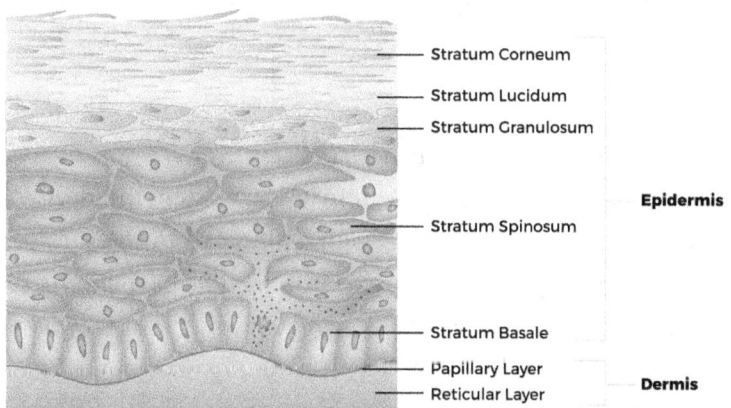

The Dermis

The dermis is the deeper of the two layers, and it is comprised of two separate layers: the *papillary* and the *reticular dermis*. The dermis contains blood vessels, roots of the hair follicles, and nerve endings that allow us to feel pain, temperature, texture, and other touch sensations. It's composed of living cells that have specific functions. If the skin is cut, the dermis is the layer that initially bleeds and then has the capacity to heal.

The Epidermis

The epidermis is the outer layer of skin, which lies on top of the dermis. Cells change as they move through the layers of the epidermis, dying as they work their way toward the outermost layer. In fact, the outermost portion of all skin is a layer of dead cells. Interestingly, toenails, fingernails, and hair are made up of dead cells. That's why cutting your hair or biting your fingernails doesn't hurt or bleed.

The epidermis is comprised of five layers, or stratum, called *stratum basale, spinosum, granulosum, lucidum,* and *corneum.*

Stratum Basale

The deepest layer is called the basal layer, or *stratum basale*. This layer connects the epidermis to the underlying dermis. This layer produces cells that migrate outward to the surface, serving as the origin of the outer skin cells. The basal layer also has pigment cells. All humans have the same skin, but they have various amounts of pigment. The level of pigment in the basal layer is the only thing that makes one person look different from another. Albinism is the complete lack of pigment cells.

We are all created equally; we simply have different amounts of pigment in our basal layer!

Stratum Spinosum

The next layer is called the spinous layer, or *stratum spinosum*. These cells produce a protein called *keratin*, which allows the skin to become nearly waterproof and gives the skin its strength and durability. The keratin ultimately ends up in the outermost layer of cells.

Stratum Granulosum

The next layer is called the granular layer, or *stratum granulosum*. These cells produce more keratin, other proteins, and lipids, which make the outer layer of the skin more waterproof.

Stratum Lucidum

The next layer of skin is present in thick skin and is called the clear layer, or *stratum lucidum*. Thick skin is located only on the bottoms of the feet and palms of the hands. These cells help reduce friction and shear forces between the granular layer and the outermost layer, giving skin additional strength.

Stratum Corneum

The outermost layer of the skin is called the *stratum corneum*. This is the layer of cells you can see and touch. They are dead cells filled with keratin, making this layer nearly waterproof. This is the first line of defense against germs entering the body. These cells slough off over time and are constantly being replaced by new ones migrating up from the deeper layers of the epidermis.

Normal skin maintains an internal balance and equilibrium. Healthy skin keeps bacteria, fungi, and all sorts of foreign debris out of the body.

Problems occur when the cells become impaired or disrupted. Dry, cracked, and damaged skin allows openings and gaps in the protective barrier. This is why it's so important to take good care of the skin all over your body and, in particular, on your feet.

Skin Examination

Question: What's the first thing you see when you look at your feet? Answer: The skin. That's also the first thing the doctor sees. Whether they realize it or not, the doctor evaluates your skin when you take off your shoes and socks, which you will now do every time you see any kind of doctor. Smooth, well-hydrated skin with no discoloration is a sign of good health. Dry, cracked, and discolored skin should generate a conversation with your doctor about the condition of your feet. Well-trained doctors look for irregularities and areas of concern. They check between the toes and look at the toenails. A visual inventory includes checking for dry skin, discolorations, irregularities, sores, growths, masses, nail issues, and more. A simple visual inspection can uncover issues that need to be addressed.

Every time you see any doctor, remove your shoes and socks, even if they don't ask you to. Always ask, "Hey doc, how do my feet look today?" You'll be amazed at the discussion that will occur because of this simple question.

Every time you see any doctor, remove your shoes and socks, even if they don't ask you to.

Temperature, Texture, and Turgor

Normal skin should be tepid to the touch, smooth, and flexible. Over time, diabetes can damage the skin and change these characteristics. Skin temperature, texture, and turgor are a reflection of one's general health and the health of the feet.

Temperature refers to how warm or cool the feet feel to the doctor, particularly when compared to each other. Ideally, each should be about the same temperature. This comparison can be helpful in a couple of ways.

A warm foot can indicate infection or inflammation. Infected areas are almost always warm to the touch. Sprains, fractures, and arthritic conditions such as gout are typically warmer. The middle of your foot is often warmer, with the bony collapse seen in Charcot foot. (Charcot foot is a very destructive process that's discussed in Chapter 8.)

A cool foot might indicate circulation issues. This is important to note if the doctor is evaluating the potential to heal from a surgical procedure, an ulcer, or an injury. A cool foot may indicate that the entire leg has very poor circulation.

Texture refers to how the surface of the skin feels, which the doctor should compare different areas of one foot to the opposite foot. Smooth skin is ideal, while rough, dry, and crusty skin is not desirable.

Turgor refers to the flexibility of the skin. Normal skin has some squishiness and give, and it can be lightly pinched between the fingers. Long-standing diabetes can change the skin from being soft and supple to firm and rubbery while taking on a shiny appearance. This is called *diabetic dermopathy*.

Dry Skin

Xerosis is the medical term for dry skin. *Marked xerosis* is excessively dry skin all over the feet. Dry skin is more common with diabetes and even more common with neuropathy. Nerves normally send impulses to millions of sweat glands to produce sweat to keep skin hydrated. With diabetic neuropathy, the nerves don't send messages to the sweat glands, and the skin isn't hydrated. Exposure to the environment also contributes to dry skin as moisture evaporates.

Dry skin initially appears as white flaky scales that may itch. Sometimes, the scales accumulate to form rock-hard sheets called *plaques*. Have you ever seen other people's crusty, dried-out heels while walking in a park, on a beach, or in a store? Now, look at your own heels. What do they look like? Dried, cracked skin on your heels is unacceptable. It must be treated.

Treatment for Dry Skin

Have you heard that you should never apply moisturizer to your feet if you have diabetes? Has anyone said that you should never put it between your toes? Hogwash! One of the best things you can do is take good care of your skin. It's crucial to the long-term management of the diabetic foot. Soft, supple, and healthy skin greatly reduces the chances of developing problems over time. Remember, always check with your foot doctor before putting anything on your feet.

We initially treat dry skin with over-the-counter topical moisturizers, applied three to four times per day. It sounds like a lot, but it's the only way to maintain the proper level of moisture in the skin. Remember, the sweat glands aren't being instructed to produce sweat, so the moisture must be preserved in other ways.

One of the best things you can do is take good care of your skin. It's crucial to the long-term management of the diabetic foot.

Furthermore, when you frequently apply moisturizer to your feet, you'll become intimately familiar with the appearance of your feet. You're more likely to notice an abnormality when you look at your feet all the time, and you can uncover issues that need to be addressed. The simple process of frequently applying inexpensive moisturizer will help prevent more costly treatment. As Benjamin Franklin once said, "An ounce of prevention is worth a pound of cure."

Moisturizers

Skin gets dry when moisture evaporates. Moisturizers are used to keep skin hydrated. Many people think moisturizers work by adding a lot of moisture into the skin. Contrary to popular belief, they don't add much moisture to the skin. Instead, they create a barrier that prevents the evaporation of the moisture already in the skin.

Moisturizers are used frequently because the barrier effect doesn't last long. In fact, it needs to be applied to the feet three to four times daily, each and every day. No exceptions. Moisturizer is the cheapest, best medicine diabetics can use to keep the skin hydrated, healthy, and in good condition.

Moisturizer is the cheapest, best medicine diabetics can use to keep the skin hydrated, healthy, and in good condition.

Moisturizers differ based on the active ingredient and the vehicle used to deliver it to the skin. The three vehicles are lotions, creams, and gels, and each has a different ability to prevent evaporation. Gels are most effective at preventing evaporation, while creams are less effective, and lotions are least effective. Gels are also soothing and are used to treat fissures. Remember, you must check with your foot doctor before putting anything on your feet.

Over-the-Counter Moisturizers

Over-the-counter moisturizers come in a variety of formulations and are marketed for all kinds of conditions. Some are marketed for general dry skin, while others are marketed for diabetes. Some are marketed for hands, while others are marketed for feet. Some are marketed for the face, while others are marketed for the elbows. Some are marketed to repair the skin, while others are marketed for sensitive skin. Is there really any difference?

These designations are simply marketing. Do you truly think hand cream can't be used on the feet? Will face moisturizer make your elbows fall off? There's not a significant difference among them. They may have different active ingredients, but each works in nearly the same way. The unique makeup of your personal chemistry is why one brand works well for you and another brand works well for someone else. There isn't one specific brand that works best for everyone. People need to try several different brands until they find the one that works best with their skin.

Prescription Moisturizers

Prescription moisturizers tend to work better than over-the-counter preparations because they also help break down the inter-cellular connections to varying degrees while providing a barrier to evaporation. They're most appropriate when treating significantly dry skin. Over-the-counter moisturizers can be used once the skin has improved with the prescription moisturizers.

Homespun Advice

There's another dry skin treatment regimen that I've found useful over the years. Apply greasy petroleum jelly to both feet four times per day for two weeks. This will dramatically improve the skin in a relatively short timeframe. After two weeks, switch to regular moisturizer, but be sure to apply it three to four times per day. Remember to check with your foot doctor first to make sure it's safe for you.

Fissures

Fissures are deep, linear cracks in the skin caused by excessively dry skin, similar to the cracks you sometimes see on dried-out lake beds. They cause pain and a burning sensation because they expose the nerves in the deeper parts of the skin. Patients with neuropathy may not know they have them because they can't feel the burning or pain. Fissures also tend to bleed from disrupted capillaries in the deeper layers of the skin. Treatment consists of applying occlusive moisturizers to aggressively hydrate the skin. Topical antibiotic gels are used to diminish infection and help the healing process.

Chapter 4

CORNS AND CALLUSES

Patients, physicians, and insurance companies think corns and calluses are trivial. They think these are minor irritations and don't warrant a lot of attention. However, this couldn't be further from the truth in the world of diabetic foot care. The mere presence of a corn or callus indicates a problem.

Most foot doctors call corns and calluses *lesions*; however, this term does not refer to cancer. The formation of any lesion is significant because it indicates long-term increased pressure on that specific part of the foot.

The mere presence of a corn or callus indicates a problem.

Corns and calluses are made of the same cells from the same outer layer of skin. Corns are generally considered to be thick and deep, while calluses are thinner and more spread out. Calluses are commonly found on the bottom of the ball of the foot, while corns are more commonly found over the prominent knuckles of hammertoes. These lesions form because of pressure on the skin.

Initially, the skin tries to protect itself by becoming thicker. Unfortunately, this creates even more pressure, and the lesions continue to thicken. This cycle repeats and repeats. Eventually, the skin becomes overwhelmed, and an ulcer forms.

Patients with neuropathy typically don't feel pain with these lesions. This is why neuropathy causes so much trouble. It's not the patient's fault that they can't feel pain. Pain is the body's way of telling us that something is wrong. The skin continues to be injured without the protection of the pain response.

When an ulcer forms on a numb foot, the patient can't feel it and often doesn't even know it's there. The ulcer gets larger and then becomes infected. This scenario is very common, and most foot doctors see this almost every day. Some ulcers deepen until the bone becomes infected. Removal of the infected bone with amputation of the toe becomes necessary.

It's no surprise that "bathroom surgery" leads to these situations. People with diabetes, neuropathy, poor circulation, poor vision, and arthritis try to treat themselves but only contribute to a destructive process. It's very important to have a foot doctor treat what seems like a simple thing. I hope you can now appreciate how something as "trivial" as a corn or callus can turn into a disaster when left untreated or mistreated. Go to the foot doctor to receive proper care.

People with diabetes, neuropathy, poor circulation, poor vision, and arthritis try to treat themselves but only contribute to a destructive process.

What Are Corns and Calluses?

Corns and calluses form in response to pressure. They are excessive accumulations of the outer skin cells.

Corns are generally shaped like pointy ice cream cones, with the point of the cone extending into the deeper levels of the skin. Many patients want to know how long the roots are and how deep they go. Contrary to many people's beliefs, corns don't have roots or tentacles that spread out beneath the skin.

Calluses are more widespread and generally lack a deep central core. Sometimes, corns are found in the middle of a callus.

Callous   Corn

Stratum Corneum

— Skin Surface —

Stratum Corneum

Corns and calluses grow as a response to pressure on the skin over time. You might think that these lesions get to a certain size, and then the cells stop accumulating. Actually, there's no "off" switch if pressure continues to be applied to the skin. These lesions can grow to impressive sizes and depths.

Direct Pressure and Sheer Pressure

There are two types of pressure that cause lesions to form: direct and sheer. To some degree, most areas of the foot are subjected to both types of pressure at all times.

Direct pressure is when something is being pressed into the skin. It could be from an external force, such as a tight-fitting shoe that presses on a toe, or from an internal force such as a bone spur that presses into the skin from below.

Sheer pressures are applied to the skin in a more indirect way as friction is created when the foot slides within the shoe.

Direct pressure causes more corns to form, while sheer pressure causes more calluses.

Where on the Foot Are Corns and Calluses Located?

Certain areas of the foot are more prone to developing corns and calluses because they're commonly exposed to increased pressure. However, lesions can form anywhere on the foot and are sometimes found in unlikely places such as beneath the arch.

Corns are more commonly found on top of one of the small toes, with the little toe being the classic location. Calluses are most often found beneath the ball of the foot.

Why Do Corns and Calluses Hurt?

Corns and calluses often cause tremendous pain, but many people don't realize that the pain is coming from these lesions. They either try to treat themselves, or they think the pain is normal.

Foot pain is not normal. The body uses pain as a way of communicating that something is wrong. If you have foot pain, you should see a foot doctor.

Corns and calluses get thicker and harder with persistent pressure; sometimes, they get as hard as a rock. They're simply layer upon layer of dead cells that contain no nerves. So, why do these nerve-free layers of dead skin cells hurt so much?

Corns and calluses hurt because they press on the nerves in the deeper layers of the skin. Some feel a burning sensation beneath the ball of the foot, while others say it feels as if the foot is on fire.

Foot pain is not normal. The body uses pain as a way of communicating that something is wrong. If you have foot pain, you should see a foot doctor.

Self-Treatment of Corns and Calluses

It's common for people to self-treat corns and calluses at home. If you were to stroll down the aisles of your favorite pharmacy, you'd see a variety of products that allegedly treat corns and calluses: non-medicated and medicated pads, metal and plastic tools, razor blades, pumice stones, mechanical grinders, liquid medications, and more.

If you have diabetes, neuropathy, and/or poor circulation, you should **never** use any of these products. If you are not sure if you have neuropathy or poor circulation, you should **never** use any of these products. Few people know how to use them properly, and the incorrect use of such products often leads to bigger problems. You must get permission from your foot doctor before using anything on your feet.

---

*If you have diabetes, neuropathy, and/or poor circulation, you should **never** use any of these products.*

Bathroom Surgery

Bathroom surgery refers to any self-care at home, even when it doesn't take place in the bathroom. It often leads to more problems than it solves. Many people cut or scrape themselves and then are unaware of the damage they have created. Don't do it! Neuropathy and/or poor circulation exacerbates these self-inflicted injuries, sometimes beyond the point of being curable. Foot doctors perform many amputations because of bathroom surgery.

Mr. Herman, who has diabetes with neuropathy and poor circulation, kept putting medicated pads on his little toe. The medicine in the pads soon burned a hole in his toe—all the way down to the bone. He thought something looked funny and decided to try to cut off the funny-looking thing sticking out of his toe. He was trying to cut off the bone that was sticking out of his toe. Mr. Herman quickly learned not to put any medicated pads on his remaining nine toes.

Mrs. Tilly, also a diabetic with neuropathy and poor circulation, was in the garage using her tin snips to cut her toenails. The dirty tool led to the infection of all the toes on her right foot. Mrs. Tilly doesn't cut the five remaining toenails on her left foot with tin snips any longer.

Instruments of Destruction

Many devices are used to perform bathroom surgery. Patients admit to using razors, scissors, tin snips, screwdrivers, pocket knives, tweezers, steak knives, and even their own fingernails. Does this sound familiar? These instruments of destruction often lead to injury and are typically dirty, dull, and completely inappropriate. Please don't do this to yourself. Go to the foot doctor.

And let's not forget that people can barely reach their feet, let alone work on them. Back, hip, and knee problems prevent people from bending over far enough to reach their feet. Poor vision prevents them from seeing what they are trying to do, and arthritic hands prevent them from manipulating the poorly chosen tools.

This creates a dangerous situation. It's no mystery why bathroom surgery leads to problems for so many patients. It's not worth the risk to do it yourself. The foot doctor has the knowledge, skills, and the right tools to manage these conditions properly.

Home Remedies

Pumice Stones

Pumice stones are medical-grade grinders used to reduce corns and calluses, available at many pharmacies and retailers without a prescription. Despite the name, a pumice stone is not a rock.

The head is either a sandpaper or cheese grater-like rasp on the end of a stick. Lesions are reduced by rubbing the pumice stone over them, with each swipe scraping off another layer of cells. Damage occurs when people try to remove too much tissue at once.

Pumice stones are not intended as initial treatment, and they are not meant to eliminate lesions. They help prevent lesions from quickly returning and are best used after the foot doctor reduces the lesions in the office. The best time to use one is when the skin is soft and supple, right after getting out of the tub or shower. However, the idea is not to "go to town" on the corn or callus.

The pumice stone has the same relationship to the corn or callus as the toothbrush does to plaque. You don't allow plaque to build up on your teeth for a couple of months and then try to get it all off at once. You brush your teeth every day and remove a little plaque each time. Similarly, the pumice stone removes a little bit of the corn or callus each day, not the whole thing all at once. Do not use a pumice stone without permission from your foot doctor.

Power Grinders

Power grinders can be difficult to control and may grind off normal skin. They can also burn the skin if left in one place for too long. If you have diabetes, poor circulation, and/or neuropathy, these devices can cause serious harm and should not be used.

Padding

Padding is used for many reasons. It's available in a nearly unlimited variety of colors, shapes, sizes, and materials. It's divided into two types: non-medicated and medicated.

Non-Medicated Padding

Non-medicated padding is applied on top of—or around—lesions and prominent bones. This makes the shoe rub on the pad, not the foot. Some are used to provide cushion beneath the ball of the foot.

Many pads come in sheets that are custom cut to fit specific contours of the foot. Donut pads come with strategically placed holes. Non-medicated padding often has an adhesive backing to help secure it in place. Patients often come into the office with pads slipped out of place. I tease them and ask, "Why don't you just staple them on?"

Moleskin

Moleskin is a thin, adhesive-backed felt-like material used to reduce sheer pressure under the ball of the foot and on the back of the heel. Despite its name, it's not actually mole skin. Available in pre-cut sizes, it's usually custom cut from large sheets to accommodate specific contours of the foot.

Tube Foam

Tube foam, as the name implies, is tube-shaped soft foam placed around individual toes. It's available in multiple sizes for different-sized toes, and some have silicone or gel linings to further reduce pressure.

Tube foam can be dangerous because it completely encircles the toe. It can strangulate a toe and completely cut off the circulation. I've seen toes become gangrenous due to tube foam. If you have diabetic neuropathy and/or poor circulation, you should not use anything that completely surrounds any toe.

Non-medicated padding reduces pressure on many parts of the foot, but it's not always safe or appropriate. Always check with your foot doctor before you put anything on your feet.

Medicated Padding:

Medicated padding has medication in or on the padding. Typically, the "medicine" is either 17 or 40 percent salicylic acid, which helps soften and reduce lesions by breaking apart the intercellular glue that holds the outer skin cells together. This frees the cells from one another and allows them to fall away. Even though this sounds great, medicated pads can be very dangerous and should never be used if you're diabetic.

The problem is that there's no regulator—or off switch—to stop the action of the medication. Furthermore, salicylic acid, as the name implies, is acid! It can break down the surrounding normal skin and create a chemical burn. That's why the medication is known to "burn away" lesions.

Another problem is that it's difficult to apply medicated pads to the lesions alone. They're often mistakenly applied to the surrounding skin that's thinner and less resistant to the action of the salicylic acid. If you have normal sensation, you'll feel the burn, know there's a problem, and hopefully remove the pads. But if you have neuropathy, you can't feel the burn, so you'll leave the medicated pad on your skin and suffer damaging side effects without realizing it.

Mr. Oscar came into the office because his wife thought something was wrong with his little toe. He'd been applying medicated pads to the toe for only a few days. When I removed the medicated pad, I saw the bone sticking out. The medication had burned away all the skin. His neuropathy prevented him from feeling the destruction, which progressed in only a few days. His wife doesn't use medicated pads on the nine toes he has left.

Toes are amputated because the person didn't appreciate the potential danger of medicated pads. If you're a diabetic, throw away all medicated pads and never use them again. Let your foot doctor take care of your lesions.

People still try to treat themselves even when they know better. I suppose the number one reason has to do with cost. But consider this: the cost of a visit to the foot doctor is almost always cheaper than the cost to treat an infection or worse in the long run.

Continue to see your foot doctor on a regular basis. Even if you don't have any problems, you should still see your foot doctor at least once per year. This greatly reduces the chances of developing problems with your feet. Be diligent about your regular visits. The sooner any problem is discovered, the more quickly treatment can begin and the less chance of major catastrophe.

Professional Treatment of Corns and Calluses

Foot doctors spend a great deal of time treating corns and calluses, and they have more experience than any other provider in treating these conditions. If you have diabetes, you need professional foot care. It's not appropriate to have a nurse or a nail salon take care of diabetic feet.

If you have diabetes, you need professional foot care.

Treatment is based upon one's medical history and lower extremity health. The medical history includes things like the current medical conditions, medications, and allergies. Many factors are examined when a doctor evaluates the lower extremities, such as determining whether there is good or bad circulation, the degree of neuropathy if present, foot deformities, skin integrity, and toenail pathology. This information is used to formulate the best treatment plan for each patient.

Both surgical and non-surgical options are available when treating corns and calluses. I like to explore the conservative treatments before I recommend surgery. Ultimately, the goal is to reduce pressure on the skin to prevent or eliminate lesions. Simply put, non-surgical treatments reduce pressure on the skin from the outside, while surgical options reduce pressure on the skin from the inside.

Non-Surgical Treatments

Foot doctors are experts at providing non-surgical treatment for corns and calluses. Treatments include debridement, padding, and appropriate shoe gear.

Debridement

Debridement is the medical term for paring down lesions with some type of blade. It reduces the lesions one layer at a time and is the most common treatment.

Foot doctors spend a great deal of time debriding lesions. It's difficult to do well, and it takes years of experience to become proficient. It's not as simple as it looks. We know when to keep going and, more importantly, when to stop. We've learned how to remove the deep little cores without harming the surrounding tissues. Good foot doctors have mastered debridement.

Sterile, sharp blades of various sizes and shapes are used to debride lesions. Sharp blades work best because they slice through the tissues easier and with more precision. Surgical scalpel blades are often used because they're sterile and very sharp.

Dull instruments used for bathroom surgery cause more damage because they drag and move poorly through the tissues. Have you noticed that you prefer the sharpest knife in the kitchen? That's because it makes cutting food a lot easier.

Sharp blades cause less damage to the surrounding tissues because they're more precise and easier to control. Occasionally, even a foot doctor will nick the surrounding skin. That's why a new, sterile blade is used for each patient.

Take note of the way your foot doctor prepares the treatment room. Is the office organized? Do the instruments appear fresh and clean? Or are the instruments dirty and strewn haphazardly around the room? Make sure that your doctor uses a new blade at every visit. Does your foot doctor look well-groomed and neat? Or is he or she sloppy and disheveled? You should feel comfortable in the treatment chair. A clean, organized treatment room is essential. If it's not, get up and leave.

Padding

Professional padding, or *orthodigita* (a term coined by Dr. Alan Whitney of Cherry Hill, New Jersey), is the art and science of creating custom padding. Generic pharmacy padding is usually more rigid and less moldable than custom padding available at the foot doctor's office. Foot doctors have access to a variety of pliable materials not available to the general public. A good foot doctor has great experience with orthodigita and knows more about custom padding than any other provider.

Appropriate Shoe Gear

Shoes are meant to protect the feet from the outside world. They should fit properly and be comfortable. I see many people wearing ill-fitting shoes that create pressure points. The foot isn't meant to be crammed into high-heeled shoes with pointy toes. Additionally, it is not meant to be stuffed into a shoe that's too small. Poorly fitting shoes lead to many problems, especially with diabetes.

    Generally speaking, a wider shoe with a taller toe box provides more room, which can greatly reduce pressure on the toes. A nice cushiony insert can reduce pressure beneath the ball of the foot, which can help eliminate calluses. Shoes should be properly fitted, particularly when neuropathy is present.

    Shoes can also be altered in strategic locations to accommodate corns and calluses and to reduce pressure on the skin. The local shoe repair shop probably has a device called the ball-and-ring that will stretch shoes to accommodate prominent areas. They create more room for the little toe when a little sidecar is stretched into the shoe. Some people cut a hole on the inside of their shoe to accommodate a large bunion or on the top of the shoe to accommodate a hammertoe that sticks up in the air. This is an easy way to manage large deformities for poor surgical candidates.

For some, wearing regular shoes is simply too uncomfortable. These patients come in wearing house slippers or sandals. Although I prefer that my patients wear a supportive shoe, the most important thing is to protect the bottom of the foot. You can wear house slippers, as long as they have a protective sole on the bottom. You don't want any foreign objects to cut, puncture, or get stuck in the bottom of your foot.

If you have diabetes, neuropathy, and/or poor circulation, you must never walk barefooted. You can't risk stepping on something that needs to be extracted from your foot. I've removed common items such as needles, thumbtacks, staples, splinters, glass, thorns, and metal shards, but I have also removed more uncommon things such as pieces of light bulbs, dog tags, pen caps, pencils, nails, and even razor blades. It's terrifying to think about the variety of items that can end up in an unprotected, numb foot.

If you have diabetes, neuropathy, and/or poor circulation, you must never walk barefooted.

Properly Fit Shoes

If a shoe is labeled as a size 8, that doesn't mean it's a size 8. Don't buy shoes based on what the label says. Years ago, a size 7 shoe was a standard size 7 shoe. But now, one manufacturer's size 7 is another manufacturer's size 5, and another's size 8 or 9 or 12! Even different styles from the same manufacturer vary in size. When you buy shoes, you must be properly fitted for each pair at a reputable shoe store.

High Heels

High heels and pointy-toed shoes are stylish but often create problems. They transfer the weight of the body forward, which increases pressure beneath the ball of the foot. Pointy-toed shoes can wreak havoc on the toes. There's no way that five toes can be scrunched into a point and not experience increased pressure and rubbing. Bunions and hammertoes are often aggravated by pointy-toed shoes. I tell my patients to wear more rounded, flatter-heeled shoes, but some don't listen. Altering the choice of the heel height and the roundedness of the toe box can make a significant difference.

Surgical Treatment of Corns and Calluses

Surgery is considered after conservative treatments fail to improve the situation. Lesions form when undue pressure is placed on the skin. Surgery reduces the pressure on the skin from prominent bones inside the foot.

Many surgical procedures are performed to reduce or eliminate corns, calluses, and ulcers. The five most common surgeries address bunions, bunionettes, hammertoes, bone spurs, and prominent bones beneath the ball of the foot.

Looks Like a Corn or Callus but Isn't

Corns and calluses have a certain look, but other conditions have a similar appearance. Patients and doctors often mistakenly treat other conditions as corns or calluses.

Warts

Warts, called verruca, are commonly mistaken for corns and calluses. They have a similar appearance because they form in the same outer layer of skin but are not caused by pressure. Warts are viral infections in the skin caused by the human papillomavirus, HPV. Humans can develop one, a few, or many at the same time. Mosaic warts are clusters of multiple small warts in one area.

It's thought that people are more susceptible to warts when the immune system doesn't fight off the virus. Children, young adults, and people with immune system deficiencies are at the most risk. Warts are contagious and should be treated as soon as possible to prevent them from spreading and because they seem to become more resistant to treatment over time.

Plantar Warts

Plantar warts, by definition, are found on the bottom of the foot. They are caused by the same HPV virus that causes other warts and not, as some think, a different type of virus. A plantar wart is like any other wart, except it's usually located beneath the ball of the foot or heel. Walking presses these warts deeper into the foot, giving them the rightful reputation of being difficult to treat.

Normal skin has ridges and whorls that are called skin lines. You may know these as fingerprints. Warts differ from normal skin by lacking skin lines, leaving no fingerprints. Corns and calluses initially have skin lines but lose them as they become thicker and more irregular.

Warts also often have little black dots, which are not present in normal skin, corns, or calluses. The black dots are little capillaries located just below the surface. When a wart is pared down with a blade, the little capillaries bleed. This is called pinpoint bleeding. Corns and calluses lack capillaries and don't bleed when pared down or debrided. However, sometimes the surrounding skin can be nicked, and that bleeds. Also, corns and calluses that have been present for a long time can disrupt the integrity of the underlying skin, leading to blood in or under a corn or callus.

Skin Cancer

Skin cancer can be mistaken for corns, calluses, or warts. Historically, skin cancer has certain characteristics that may or may not be present, including a lesion that changes size; bleeds easily; has irregular borders; is colored red, white, or blue; or is darkly pigmented. Lesions with any of these characteristics are suspicious and must be evaluated.

However, these are generalities and not absolute. Not all skin cancers follow these rules. Many non-cancerous lesions have some of these same characteristics. Unfortunately, the reverse is also true. Many skin cancers have none of those characteristics. In fact, clear cell skin cancer, as the name implies, lacks many of these characteristics.

Lesions with any of these characteristics are suspicious and must be evaluated.

I've often had people come to my office after years of self-treatment for a corn that wouldn't go away. Unfortunately, the lesion turned out to be skin cancer, which is why all lesions need to be examined by a foot doctor, internist, or dermatologist. The earlier skin cancer is identified, the better the outcome.

Ingrown toenails

Any discussion of skin cancer on the foot must include infected ingrown toenails. The medical term for this is *paronychia*. Patients were treated by removing the ingrown toenail, multiple courses of antibiotics, foot soaks, and topical antibiotic creams. The toe improved for a while but would always worsen again or simply never heal.

Patients can visit several offices with this story. A subsequent doctor becomes suspicious because the "infection" never went away. A biopsy would confirm the presence of skin cancer and not infection. Frequently, amputation of the toe and evaluation by an oncologist (cancer doctor) is necessary.

Clogged Sweat Glands

Porokeratosis is a clogged sweat gland that resembles a corn or callus. Sweat glands are sacs—or pockets—that extend into the deeper layers of the skin. The walls of the sac are made of the same cell layers as the outside skin. When the top of the sweat gland is clogged, the cells inside the sac become trapped and can't fall away. The cells then concentrate into a hard, deep, corn-like growth in the skin.

Treatment involves debriding the lesion to open the sac and remove the buildup of cells. Sometimes, we freeze clogged sweat glands to get rid of the entire growth. Foot doctors are very familiar with porokeratosis.

Many lesions resemble corns and calluses. All lesions should be evaluated by a foot doctor or dermatologist. Although tempting, people should not work on these by themselves, particularly those with diabetes, neuropathy, and/or poor circulation.

Chapter 5

DIABETES AND CIRCULATION

Sufficient blood flow is essential for healthy feet. Cells receive vital nutrients and oxygen from the blood. Reduced blood flow diminishes the cell's ability to function properly and prevents healing factors from reaching damaged areas. Poor healing is often due to poor blood flow to the area. Most know that circulation diminishes with age. Diabetes causes the circulation to deteriorate quicker and at an earlier age.

Diabetes affects the circulation down the entire lower extremity, which includes the thigh, knee, calf, ankle, foot, and toes. The leg includes the calf and shin and is the part of the lower extremity only between the knee and ankle. The thigh is above the knee. Poor circulation to the toes often means there is poor circulation down the entire lower extremity. Think about that for a minute. It's less common for the blood flow to be fine through the thigh, knee, calf, ankle, and foot, and then all of a sudden, it's poor to only the toes. Usually, it's poor all the way down the entire lower extremity.

The primary reason for poor healing is reduced blood flow. Complete lack of blood flow leads to tissue death, or gangrene, and amputation.

Let's suppose a diabetic patient comes in with a gangrenous, dead toe. There's no hope of saving that toe, and it needs to be amputated. We need to appreciate that this person probably has poor circulation above his or her toe as well. We must find out how bad the circulation is throughout the rest of the lower extremity. We wouldn't want to amputate the toe and then find out that poor circulation prevents the incision from healing. The next level would be amputated, and since the circulation through that level is also poor, it doesn't heal either. You'd end up with progressive amputations of more and more of the foot and eventually the leg.

We want to avoid this "chop, chop, chop." We want to determine the best course of treatment in the beginning, based upon the circulation to the whole lower extremity. It sometimes makes more sense to amputate more of the foot than one might think necessary, so the remainder of the foot has the best chance to heal.

Evaluating Circulation

Evaluating the circulation throughout the whole lower extremity is critical when it comes to the diabetic foot. It provides better insight into the healing potential of the foot and better management of complex situations.

Circulation to the lower extremities is evaluated in several ways. The first way is for the foot doctor to look at the feet. The overall appearance gives a general, rudimentary picture of how good or bad the circulation may be.

Healthy, smooth, supple skin with no marks or discolorations suggests the circulation is good. Discolored, tight, and shiny skin suggests it may be poor. However, appearances can be deceiving. Good-looking skin may have poor circulation, and unhealthy appearing skin may have great circulation. The only way to determine the actual circulation is with testing.

Peripheral arterial disease, or PAD, is an abnormality of the arteries that leads to reduced circulation to the lower extremity. You may have seen commercials for medicines that treat PAD. These advertisements make it sound like PAD is a new disease that's just been discovered. It isn't. The term PAD has been used by foot doctors and vascular surgeons for decades. But recently, new treatments have come forward, and the publicity of the condition has increased.

Pulses

We can feel blood flow through an artery with our fingertips as the artery expands and contracts with each heartbeat. There is a pulse point in the wrist, two in the neck, and one in front of each ear. Feeling a pulse with the fingertips is called *palpating a pulse.*

Normally, there are two pulse points on each foot. One is on top of the foot, and the other is behind the inside of the ankle. The pulse on top of the foot is called the *dorsalis pedis pulse,* which is Latin for "top of the foot." The one behind the inner ankle is called the *posterior tibial pulse,* which is Latin for "behind the ankle bone."

Pulses are graded in terms of how strong they feel when palpated. A strong pulse is easily palpated and suggests adequate circulation. A weak pulse is more difficult to feel and suggests reduced circulation. We have a system that describes the strength of the pulse, ranging from 0/4, which is very poor, to 4/4, which is extremely strong.

- 0/4 pulse can't be felt and is called "non-palpable."
- 1/4 pulse can be felt but is weak.
- 2/4 pulse can be felt without difficulty and is considered normal.
- 3/4 pulse is strong and easy to feel.
- 4/4 pulse can be seen pulsating through the skin and is very strong.[6]

Non-Palpable Pulses and Good Circulation

Non-palpable pulses usually reflect poor circulation. However, circulation can be adequate even with non-palpable pulses.

Normally, the walls of each artery are made of flexible, elastic muscle. You can feel the pulse of normal arteries when the muscle wall is expanded by the blood passing through with each heartbeat. Calcification of the muscular wall makes the artery hard and inelastic. The medical term for this is *arteriosclerosis* or *hardening of the arteries*. Blood still passes through the patent

---

[6] Hill, R. Dean, Smith, Robert B. III, "Examination of the Extremities: Pulses Bruits, and Phlebitis." In: *Clinical Methods: The History, Physical, and Laboratory Examinations*, 3rd edition, ed Walker, H. K.; Hall, W.D.; Hurst, J. W., (Boston: Butterworths: 1990), https://pubmed.ncbi.nlm.nih.gov/21250191/.

center, even though the artery doesn't expand, and the pulse cannot be felt. In long-standing diabetes, calcified arteries can actually be seen on X-ray images.

Palpable Pulses and Poor Circulation

Sometimes, the pulse is strong, but the circulation to a toe is bad. This happens when the larger arteries are elastic and patent, but the tiny blood vessels to the toes, called *capillaries*, are blocked. Ironically, a very strong pulse is sometimes palpable right next to an area of dead tissue or gangrene.

Blockages within a large artery often cause reduced circulation to the lower extremity. These usually form in the thigh, around the knee, and in the leg. They're due to a gradual buildup of fat in the arteries. This is called *atherosclerosis*. Vascular surgeons frequently perform bypass surgery around these blockages to restore blood flow to the foot.

Photoplethysmography

Photoplethysmography (PPG) is used to determine blood flow and oxygen levels in the capillaries of the toes and fingers. This is the monitor they put on your finger when you have surgery. PPG works by sending a painless light into the skin. The levels of blood flow and oxygen reflect the light back to the PPG. This information is then converted to waveforms. Better blood flow displays as higher waveforms, while oxygen concentrations are expressed as percentages. Low waveforms indicate poor circulation, and low percentages reflect less oxygenation to the tissues. All hospitals and surgery centers keep these devices on your finger to make sure your blood flow is good and your tissues are receiving proper oxygen levels during surgery. Most doctor offices don't have these devices unless they frequently provide in-depth vascular exams.

Doppler Studies

We use Doppler studies to evaluate the circulation when pulses can't be palpated. The Doppler is a pencil-shaped stick with a transducer and microphone located at the tip. The transducer sends painless, inaudible ultrasonic sound waves through the skin to the arteries. The sound waves bounce off the blood flow in the artery being tested and are sent back to the microphone on the tip of the Doppler. The sound waves received by the microphone are then amplified to a speaker.

The better the blood flow, the louder the pulsation can be heard on the speaker. You can easily hear the pulsations as the Doppler is applied over an artery with good circulation. Less is heard with poor circulation, as fewer sound waves reflect back to the Doppler. These studies are very good at demonstrating adequate circulation when the pulses are not palpable.

Doppler studies can determine that blood flow through a particular artery is poor, but it does not identify where the blockage is located.

Non-Invasive Vascular Evaluation and Arteriogram

There are two tests that can identify the location of a blockage. The non-invasive vascular evaluation (NIVE) is performed in an office. It is comprised of several tests, including the ankle-brachial index, segmental pressures, and waveforms.

Ankle-Brachial Index

The ankle-brachial index (ABI) gives a general overview of the circulation to the foot. It compares the blood pressure at the ankle to the blood pressure in the arm. Circulation to the foot is probably good if the blood pressure at the ankle closely compares to the blood pressure in the arm.

ABI is reported as a decimal, which reflects the relationship of the ankle blood pressure to the arm blood pressure. When the blood pressures are identical, the ABI is 1.0. If the ankle blood pressure is lower than the arm, the ABI would be less than 1.0. Suppose the ankle blood pressure is half the blood pressure in the arm, the ABI would be 0.5. Conversely, if the ankle blood pressure were 25 percent higher than the arm, the ABI would be 1.25. An ABI of 0.9 to 1.3 is considered normal. An ABI of 0.4 to 0.9 suggests mild to moderate peripheral arterial disease, and an ABI less than 0.4 suggests severe peripheral arterial disease.

Segmental Pressures

Segmental pressures compare blood pressures of multiple levels of one lower extremity to each other and to the other lower extremity. This part of the NIVE is easy to perform and very important. It involves placing multiple blood pressure cuffs at the thigh, leg, foot, and toes of both lower extremities. Blood pressure cuffs are available in a variety of sizes, including a very small one that is wrapped around the big toe. A Doppler is used to hear the return of blood flow as the cuffs are inflated and deflated in a specific order.

The results of the circulation test are broken down in several ways. The first portion of the test determines the blood pressure at different levels of each lower extremity. These recordings, measured in millimeters of mercury (mmHg), are compared to the arm blood pressure, as well as to each other. Blood pressures similar to each other reflect normal circulation. A significant decrease from one level to the next suggests a blockage between those two levels. Generally speaking, a drop of 50 mmHg between two consecutive levels is considered significant.

Interestingly, a significant increase in blood pressure from one level to the next also suggests a problem, as the blood flow hits a partial blockage and raises the blood pressure. This phenomenon is similar to putting your thumb over the end of a garden hose.

Waveforms

The second aspect of the NIVE compares waveforms created using the blood pressure cuffs and the Doppler. The blood pressure cuffs are inflated and deflated with the Doppler device placed over an artery in the foot. As the various blood pressure cuffs are inflated, the blood flow is temporarily stopped. As the cuff is deflated, blood flow returns past that particular cuff. The Doppler measures the intensity of the returning blood flow, which is graphed with a waveform. Higher intensity means better blood flow and a higher waveform.

Conversely, poor circulation creates flattened waveforms on the graphs. A significantly flatter waveform immediately following a good waveform suggests the location of the blockage.

Waveforms are evaluated independently and in comparison to other levels. Sudden flattening of a waveform is significant. Flattening of most of the waveforms indicates poor circulation throughout the entire lower extremity.

Interpretation of the NIVE

NIVE data is used to evaluate the circulation and locate blockages in order to tailor appropriate treatment. Ask your doctor to review the report with you. You will learn a lot about your circulation.

Arteriogram

The arteriogram is the second test used to determine the exact location of a blockage. It is the gold standard of vascular testing because it's the best way to demonstrate the actual circulation to the entire lower extremity. It is performed in the vascular lab at the hospital by a radiologist and interpreted by the vascular surgeon. It involves injecting a special dye into the arteries, which can then be seen on X-ray images.

The arteriogram identifies the exact location and size of arterial blockages. The X-ray images create a map of the blood flow from the hip to the toes. Normal or near-normal circulation shows the dye traveling all the way down to the toes without interruption. The dye will suddenly stop at the level of a complete blockage, and it thins at the level of a partial blockage.

Blockages can be opened or completely bypassed by vascular surgeons to improve or restore circulation to the lower extremity and foot. This is often performed to help heal ulcers and prevent amputation.

Reba went to see her internist because she had a funny smell coming from her foot. The internist knew the foot was infected, so Reba was sent to the foot doctor. The foot doctor took some X-rays of the foot and discovered the infection was in the bone. Reba was admitted to the hospital, where her blood sugar level was over 400 mg%. Reba's diabetes was out of control, and she had a nasty foot infection. The foot doctor couldn't feel pulses in her feet, so a Doppler was ordered. The Doppler showed poor circulation, and the foot doctor knew he had to amputate part of the foot. In order to evaluate the true nature of the circulation to the entire lower extremity, a non-invasive vascular evaluation was ordered. The test showed that Reba actually had pretty decent circulation down most of the lower extremity but poor circulation from the middle of the foot to her toes.

The foot doctor knew that removing only the front part of the foot would likely heal with good control of her diabetes. The vascular surgeon, infectious disease doctor, and foot doctor were able to save Reba's leg and most of her foot. Reba now wears a shoe filler where her toes were.

This story is repeated every day in many hospitals across America. Reba now takes better care of her diabetes and pays attention to her feet.

Circulation

Arteries are the pipes that carry blood from the heart to the organs of the body and feet. Veins are the pipes that return the blood back to the heart from the organs of the body and the feet. Blood cycles through the lungs to get a fresh supply of oxygen. It's a process that continues with each heartbeat.

Blood flow can be interrupted in the arteries and veins. Arterial blockages are usually caused by a buildup of fat, while venous blockages are mostly caused by blood clots.

Arterial Blockages

Atherosclerosis is the buildup of fat inside an artery that inhibits or prevents blood flow. It most commonly occurs in the artery in the thigh, called the *femoral artery*. A piece of the fatty blockage may break off and travel down the artery. The piece of fat traveling down the artery is called an embolus. The process is called an embolic event.

Emboli lodge in the smaller arteries and inhibit or prevent circulation past that point. Some create little black spots on the toes, which are small patches of gangrene. This indicates that some of the fatty blockage has broken off and traveled down to the foot. Even though these black spots usually heal over time, it's important to recognize the presence of a blockage somewhere higher up. Determining the size and location of the blockage is important.

Venous Blockages

Venous blockages are usually due to the buildup of platelets inside the vein. Pieces of venous blood clots that break off travel to the heart and lungs, not the feet. An arterial embolic event may lead to the death of a toe, but it won't kill you. Pulmonary embolism (PE) occurs when part of a blood clot in a vein travels to the lungs. The sudden loss of circulation to the lungs makes it difficult to breathe and quickly becomes life-threatening.

Most pulmonary emboli break off from clots in the deep veins of the calf. These are known as deep vein thrombosis (DVT). Recognizing DVT is critical in order to prevent death. DVT occurs after surgery when patients are more sedentary. Many are prescribed blood thinners after surgery to prevent DVT. Some have an umbrella-type filter placed in the main chest vein to prevent sudden death when chronic DVT is present in the thigh or calf.

Circulation Medications

Circulation medicines are prescribed to prevent blood clots in the arteries and veins. Blood thinners are used to thin the blood to allow it to pass blockages in the arteries. Anticoagulants are used to prevent blood clots from forming in the veins. Some medicines help improve poor circulation.

The internist, family physician, or vascular surgeon is the doctor who usually prescribes these medicines. Some need ongoing monitoring, and most interact with other medicines. Dosages are adjusted, and sometimes, other medicines become more appropriate.

Aspirin

Aspirin thins the blood and is well known for its ability to prevent heart attacks and strokes. It can also improve circulation to the feet by helping blood flow past partial blockages in the arteries.

Aspirin acts as a blood thinner by interfering with the function of platelets. The medical term for platelet is *thrombocyte* which is Greek for "clot cell." Platelets stick together after an injury to form a plug in the skin to stop bleeding. These are "good" blood clots. We would all bleed to death each time we were cut if it weren't for platelets acting like a cork.

Venous blood clots form when platelets stick together, and the enlarging collection of platelets inhibits blood flow. Aspirin helps by preventing the platelets from sticking together and forming a clot.

Fortunately, aspirin doesn't totally prevent platelets from adhering to one another. It just takes longer. It's enough to help prevent blood clots yet still allow bleeding to eventually stop.

Trental

Trental, generic name *pentoxifylline*, is an oral medication that helps improve circulation. We don't fully understand the exact way it works, but it's thought to increase the flexibility of the red and white blood cells, allowing them to squeeze past blockages in the arteries. It's used infrequently because other medicines have replaced it.

Coumadin

Coumadin, generic name *warfarin*, is an oral medication that prevents blood clots in the veins. It prevents the liver from producing clotting factors, which depend upon vitamin K. It once was the most frequently prescribed anticoagulant, but other medicines with fewer concerns have started to replace it.

The effect of warfarin is difficult to control due to varying amounts of vitamin K in a person's diet. Increased levels of vitamin K in the diet lowers the effect of warfarin. Reduced levels of vitamin K allow warfarin to thin the blood. The problem is that the function of warfarin can go up and down each day as the intake of vitamin K varies.

The variability of warfarin therapy requires frequent monitoring. That's why if you take warfarin, you are continually tested to see how thin your blood has become. Although the test is known as "checking the Coumadin level," it's actually the degree to which the blood has been thinned by the drug that's being determined, not the level of the drug in the blood.

The blood is usually evaluated every two to four weeks. If it's found to be on the thinner side, the dose of warfarin is reduced. If the blood is not as thin as the doctor would like, the dose is increased. The blood is then reevaluated in a few weeks, and adjustments are made accordingly. Frequent monitoring and adjusting the dose is common. If you or someone you love is on warfarin, you're already familiar with this never-ending process.

The International Normalized Ratio (INR) is the primary way to determine the effectiveness of warfarin, a test formerly known as the prothrombin test (PT). The INR is evaluated as frequently as every couple of days during initial therapy or when control is difficult to maintain to about every month or so when control seems to be consistent.

The INR measures how long it takes for the blood to clot inside a test tube, compared to the time that a control sample takes to clot. A comparison between the two times determines the INR. If the sample takes longer to clot than the control sample, the INR level is a higher number, and the blood is considered to be relatively thinner. If the sample clots more quickly than the control sample, the INR is a lower number, and the blood is considered to be not as thin.

In most cases, the blood is thinned to an INR of about 2.0 to 3.0. This means the patient's blood should take two to three times longer to clot than the control sample, which usually takes between eleven to sixteen seconds. Ongoing INR monitoring allows the doctor to keep the blood thinned to the right degree, which helps prevent heart attack, stroke, and blood clots. Thinning the blood also helps improve circulation to the feet.

A dangerous situation can occur if the blood gets too thin and the INR gets too high. Bleeding easily occurs even without injury. People develop spontaneous nosebleeds or find blood in their stool from bleeding stomach ulcers. They bruise easily from simple little bumps. More importantly, the bleeding can be difficult to stop.

Sometimes, the warfarin effect needs to be reversed—and quickly. And guess what is used: vitamin K.

Plavix®

Plavix, generic name *clopidogrel*, is an oral medication that prevents blood clots in the veins by preventing platelets from sticking together. Unlike aspirin, the effect of clopidogrel on the platelets is irreversible. The platelet is permanently altered and can't bind to other platelets.

The lifespan of a platelet is about seven days. Clopidogrel must be stopped about five days prior to surgery so enough new and unaffected platelets are present during and after surgery. Clopidogrel is resumed once surgery is completed.

Eliquis®

Eliquis, generic name *apixaban*, is an oral medication that inhibits the formation of a protein critical to forming clots. It's commonly used to reduce the risk of stroke and to prevent pulmonary embolism (with a certain type of elevated heart rate called atrial fibrillation) and DVT.

Heparin

Heparin is used to prevent the formation of new blood clots and to prevent the extension of existing blood clots. It's a blood thinner given by intravenous access (I.V.) or injection under the skin. Since its blood-thinning action only lasts about one hour, it's often given through a continuous, controlled infusion. The effect is frequently monitored, and the dose can be adjusted as needed.

Heparin thins the blood in more than one way, but the primary way it works is by preventing a protein called fibrin from forming clots. Fibrin is stored in multi-fibrin packets called *fibrinogen*. Fibrin can't cause clots when it's stored in packets. When individual fibrin units are released from fibrinogen, they stick together to form clots. The protein that breaks the fibrinogen down into individual fibrin units is called *thrombin*. Heparin inhibits the action of thrombin and prevents fibrin units from being released.

Heparin also prevents blood clots by increasing the effectiveness of another protein called *antithrombin*, which also interferes with the action of thrombin. Heparin increases the function of antithrombin by more than one thousand times, essentially supercharging the antithrombin. This dramatically increased potency leads to a significant reduction in the ability to form clots.

Lovenox

Lovenox, generic name *enoxaparin*, is injected under the skin and is also known as low molecular-weight heparin. It prevents blood clots in a similar way to heparin by increasing the effectiveness of antithrombin, preventing the breakdown of fibrinogen into individual fibrin units.

Blood clots frequently form after surgery as people become sedentary and the extremities are immobilized. Enoxaparin is frequently used to prevent DVT after surgery.

Pradaxa®

Pradaxa, generic name *dabigatran,* is another oral medication that inhibits the function of thrombin. Thrombin acts to break down the multi-unit groups of fibrinogen into fibrin, which stick together to form blood clots. Dabigatran is used to help prevent blood clots and reduce the risk of stroke in patients who have atrial fibrillation.

Dabigatran has two distinct advantages over other medications. First, unlike heparin or enoxaparin, it's an oral medication, so no I.V. administration or injection is necessary. Second, unlike warfarin, frequent monitoring of the blood isn't necessary.

Xarelto®

Xarelto, generic name *rivaroxaban*, is an oral medication that inhibits the enzyme that creates thrombin, which also ultimately prevents the breakdown of fibrinogen into the individual fibrin units. It also works by inhibiting another component of the clotting system called *Factor Xa*. These two mechanisms help reduce the incidence of stroke, DVT, and pulmonary embolism, particularly in the presence of atrial fibrillation.

Brilinta®

Brilinta, generic name *ticagrelor*, is an oral medication that prevents the activation of platelets. It's used to reduce the chances of a second heart attack and stroke.

Pletal®

Pletal, generic name *cilostazol*, is an oral medication that improves blood flow to the feet. It's a *vasodilator*, which means it helps open the arteries to the feet. *Intermittent claudication* occurs when you get cramping or pain in the calf when trying to walk a distance. Cilostazol is often used to help reduce symptoms of intermittent claudication, so it helps people walk further without pain.

Chapter 6

NEUROPATHY

Neuropathy is the condition in which nerve function is impaired. It's caused by many conditions not related to diabetes, such as infection, exposure to heavy metals, alcoholism, and a multitude of medical conditions.

There are three nerve systems in the body. The first group of nerves, *the autonomic nervous system*, controls involuntary functions like breathing, heartbeat, digestion, and others. The second group, *the central nervous system*, includes only the brain and spinal cord. The third group, *the peripheral nervous system*, includes all other nerves extending from the central nervous system. These are the nerves that allow us to move, stand, walk, lift, grasp, blink, chew, feel, and more. Diabetic neuropathy affects each of these systems, but it's the effect on the peripheral nerves that result in so many problems with the feet.

Diabetic Peripheral Neuropathy

Diabetic peripheral neuropathy (DPN) is the most common type of neuropathy that affects the feet. Symptoms vary and may include tingling, numbness, shooting, burning, and a diminished ability to perceive pain. It does not cause a total absence of feeling. Some people develop an exaggerated response and become hypersensitive, while others only experience pain. The inability to perceive pain is a significant concern because injuries go unnoticed and untreated.

Diabetic peripheral neuropathy (DPN) is the most common type of neuropathy that affects the feet.

How Do Nerves Work?

Nerves conduct electrical impulses from one part of the body to another. Each nerve is comprised of many individual nerve fibers, and each fiber can only transmit an impulse in one direction. Within each nerve, impulses are traveling in both directions because individual fibers run both ways. *Motor nerve fibers* transmit impulses to the muscles. This allows us to move, make a fist, chew, and walk. *Sensory nerve fibers* transmit impulses in the opposite direction to the brain. They allow us to feel things like texture, heat, cold, and pain.

Microscopically, each nerve fiber is similar to an electric wire in both structure and function. Both transmit electrical impulses along a central filament protected by an outer covering. The central part of the nerve is the *axon,* which functions like the copper filament of a wire. Surrounding the axon is a cell layer called *myelin,* which insulates the axon like the rubber coating around a copper wire.

Imagine how poorly a wire would work if the surrounding rubber were damaged or removed. The insulation would be lost, and the wire could not function properly. The impulse traveling down the wire would be interrupted, reduced, inconsistent, and sometimes not transmitted at all. Such a wire would be said to have a "short circuit." The same is true for a nerve when the myelin is damaged or removed. Symptoms of neuropathy are experienced because of the poor transmission of the impulse along the nerve fibers. The short circuit of the nerve is why people experience tingling, burning, and reduced pain perception with diabetic peripheral neuropathy.

Why Does Neuropathy Occur?

DPN tends to get worse over time as the nerves are subjected to more and more damage. The exact cause of DPN is not completely understood, and there doesn't seem to be one specific cause. However, elevated glucose levels certainly seem to play a role. It's likely that the nerves become physically damaged from a combination of three theories:

1. The *glycosylation theory* refers to high levels of glucose that physically damage the nerve cells.
2. The *microvascular theory* refers to interrupted circulation to the nerves.
3. The *polyol theory* refers to the altered metabolism of the nerves from too much sugar.

Wouldn't it be great if DPN could be treated with glucose control? Unfortunately, ideal glucose control doesn't cure or prevent neuropathy, but it does slow down its progression and helps minimize symptoms. Although we don't know all the factors that lead to DPN, we do know that uncontrolled glucose levels aggravate DPN. Patients experience exacerbated symptoms of burning, tingling, light-headedness, and even pain when glucose levels remain elevated. This is why it's so important for people to maintain appropriate glucose control.

Unfortunately, ideal glucose control won't cure or prevent neuropathy, but it may slow down its progression.

Neuropathy Medications

Neuropathy medications are used to manage neuropathy. Notice I said they *manage* neuropathy. I wish I could tell you they cure neuropathy, but they don't. They're used to reduce the symptoms of neuropathy, and we don't completely understand how they work. Some people receive great benefit from them, while others receive limited to no benefit. That's why each medicine must be tried for a period of time to see if it helps. If one doesn't offer much benefit, another is tried. Sometimes we try multiple medications until we find the right one that works for each patient.

Lyrica

Lyrica, generic name *pregabalin*, appears to help interfere with pain signals. It's commonly used for DPN and fibromyalgia.

Neurontin®

Neurontin, generic name *gabapentin*, appears to attenuate pain by acting on calcium channels along the nerves. It's used for DPN, epilepsy, and post-herpetic neuralgia.

Elavil®

Elavil, generic name *amitryptiline*, is only available as the generic in the United States. The drug appears to inhibit the uptake of certain chemicals by the nerves. It's used for DPN and depression.

Pamelor®

Pamelor, generic name *nortriptyline*, appears to inhibit the uptake of certain chemicals by the nerves. It's mostly used to treat depression but is occasionally used to treat DPN.

Metanx®

Metanx, a prescription medical food comprised of multiple vitamins, appears to improve circulation to the nerves in cases of documented *hyperhomocysteinemia*—a medical condition characterized by an abnormally high level of homocysteine in the blood. Metanx helps improve the function of cells located along the lining of blood vessels that supply blood flow to nerves. The improved circulation allows nerves to function better.

Capsaicin

Capsaicin is a topical medicine applied to the skin. It reduces substance P—a neuropeptide that acts as a neurotransmitter—

which sends pain messages to the brain. Capsaicin is the same chemical that causes the burn when you eat hot peppers.

Xylocaine®

Xylocaine, generic name *lidocaine*, is a local anesthetic. It's available in patches that are applied to the skin. It helps reduce the firing of pain fibers in the skin. It's used for DPN, generalized arthritic pain, and post-herpetic neuralgia.

Ibuprofen

Ibuprofen, most common trade names Advil® and Motrin®, is a non-steroidal, anti-inflammatory medication that helps reduce inflammation and pain. It's available in both prescription and over-the-counter strength.

Acetaminophen

Acetaminophen, most common trade name Tylenol®, reduces pain and fever but is not an anti-inflammatory.

TENS Units

TENS units, or transcutaneous electrical nerve stimulators, are battery-operated devices that deliver subtle electrical currents to the skin. They appear to stimulate sensory nerves to alleviate pain and are used for chronic pain syndromes, post-operative pain management, and occasionally for DPN.

Chapter 7

INSERTS, ARCH SUPPORTS, CUSTOM ORTHOTICS, AND CUSTOM SHOES

Inserts, arch supports, and custom orthotics are devices placed in the shoes to support and protect the foot. In the past, most inserts were called *arch supports*. Note that there's a big difference between over-the-counter inserts and custom orthotics. Inserts and arch supports are pre-made devices that don't mirror the specific contours of each foot. They're available without a prescription at many stores and local pharmacies. Custom orthotics, however, require a prescription, and they mirror the unique contours of each foot. Custom orthotics are fabricated at special laboratories from custom casts that the foot doctor takes of each foot.

Inserts, arch supports, and orthotics are used for many conditions that have nothing to do with diabetes. These include flat feet, heel pain, high arches, arthritis, generalized foot pain, neuroma, and any deformity with a bony prominence such as a bone spur, hammertoe, or bunion.

Diabetes-related conditions that require inserts or orthotics include ulcers, Charcot foot, previous amputation of part of the foot, neuropathy with poor circulation, and any deformity with a bony prominence such as a bone spur, hammertoe, or bunion. The goal is to prevent ulcers by reducing pressure on the skin.

The Trifecta of Diabetes

The trifecta of diabetes is a three-component condition that leads to ulcers that become difficult to heal. The three components are a bony prominence, peripheral neuropathy, and poor circulation. The first component is when a prominent bone rubs on the shoe. The second part—neuropathy—means patients can't feel pressure on the skin. Eventually, the skin breaks down, and an ulcer forms. The third part is when the body can't deliver the necessary healing components to a damaged area due to poor circulation.

Inserts or orthotics are mandatory for patients with this trifecta, even if they have no ulcers. The goal is to prevent ulcers from forming in the first place or to prevent them from returning once healed.

Over-the-Counter (OTC) Inserts

OTC inserts can be purchased at many stores and do not require a prescription. Prefabricated inserts, or *prefabs*, come in various sizes and shapes and are made from a variety of materials. They typically extend from the bottom of the heel to beneath the arch, with some extending beneath the ball of the foot. Full-length inserts extend to the tips of the toes and can be cut to fit the shoe. OTC inserts are available in four varieties:

"Thinserts"

The first and most basic OTC insert is generally a thin, flat inlay with no arch support. Most inserts of this type offer very little cushion and are available at almost every pharmacy. The package that contains the insert is almost as thick as the insert itself. I don't see much need for this type of insert unless there are no foot problems, no diabetes, and someone is only looking for minimal cushioning for the shoes.

Inserts with Cushion

The second type of OTC insert is more substantial and cushions the bottom of the foot, typically providing minimal-to-no arch support. They are often made from gel-based or rubber-foam materials of different densities. They provide cushion for metatarsalgia and for people who work on concrete or other hard surfaces.

Some Arch Support

The third type of OTC insert is structurally more significant. These inserts are made from multiple materials and are firmer than gel or foam. They have some type of formal arch support and are available at almost every pharmacy. Some have a generic plastic arch support beneath a soft overlay. Sometimes, the arch support is made of the cushiony material. Generic OTC arch supports are not customized to any foot.

Semi-Custom Arch Supports

Lastly, the most supportive type of OTC insert is the semi-custom insert. These are made from multiple materials and are available at many retailers.

One style comes with a variety of plastic pieces that are placed into the top of the insert to vary the arch height. Patients simply choose which one feels best. Obviously, this is not appropriate with significant deformity or with neuropathy as the prominent pieces would press into the bottom of the foot.

Another type of semi-custom insert is recommended by a computer, based on the pressure pattern created when standing on a pressure plate. The problem is that the pressure pattern of a collapsed foot may significantly differ from the pattern in the supported position.

This is particularly important with diabetes and peripheral neuropathy. The feet are in a collapsed position as the computer determines the pressure patterns. It doesn't make sense to recommend a pair of pre-made inserts based upon the pressure map of collapsed feet.

Despite some of their names, these are not custom-made orthotics. They do not take into account the subtleties and exact contours of each foot. Furthermore, they do not obtain the pressure pattern of the feet with the feet in the supported position.

If you have diabetes, peripheral neuropathy, or poor circulation, you need custom-made orthotics that are made from custom cast impressions of your feet while they are in the supported position. They are only available in a well-trained foot doctor's office.

Where Do I Buy Inserts?

A variety of retailers sell inserts. Pharmacies and medical supply stores sell inserts. Outdoor and sporting goods stores sell inserts. Chiropractors and physical therapists sell inserts. Some stores sell only inserts. Infomercials sell inserts. You can buy inserts at the hardware store. Bait shops in the middle of nowhere sell inserts. There is no training or certification required to sell most inserts. So, the obvious question is, "Where should I buy over-the-counter inserts?"

A good foot doctor's office is the best place to find out whether an OTC insert or a custom-made pair of orthotics is your best option. No other provider has more training and experience with these matters. Since safety is the first priority, don't put any inserts in your shoes without permission from your foot doctor. This may prevent injury and help avoid wasting time and money on inserts that are inappropriate. People with diabetes, foot deformity, poor circulation, or peripheral neuropathy almost always require custom orthotics.

People with diabetes, foot deformity, poor circulation, or peripheral neuropathy almost always require custom orthotics.

Custom-Made Orthotics

Custom-made orthotics require a prescription and are fabricated from individual cast impressions of each foot. They are made from a variety of materials that accommodate the specific contours and variations of each foot. As no two feet are exactly alike, no two custom orthotics are the same, even for the same person.

Non-Diabetes-Related Custom Orthotics

Custom orthotics are frequently fabricated for many non-diabetes-related conditions. This includes heel pain, flat feet, and a host of other conditions. Most of these inserts are made of high technology plastic to support the arch with some type of cushiony top cover. The level of give is determined by the foot doctor, and additional accommodations are added as needed. Some believe that nearly everyone can benefit from custom orthotics.

Diabetes-Related Custom Orthotics

Custom orthotics are most commonly prescribed to protect the feet and prevent ulceration. They are often made from softer, more forgiving materials to cushion and protect bony prominences and greatly reduce pressure. Sometimes, they are designed to provide more rigid support if needed while at the same time providing accommodation and cushion in more vulnerable areas. Some foot deformities can be quite dramatic and require bulky and wide orthotics that only fit in custom-made shoes.

Where Are Custom Orthotics Made?

Many patients want to know if foot doctors make orthotics themselves. The quick answer is no; most foot doctors do not make the orthotics themselves. All the pertinent information and appropriate accommodations are written on a prescription that is sent, along with the custom cast impressions of both feet, to an orthotic laboratory. The work required to manufacture a quality custom orthotic involves a methodical and detailed process, and it is much more involved than you would think. Simply put, most busy foot doctors don't have the time to manufacture quality custom orthotics. But they do have long-standing relationships with quality orthotic labs.

How Are Impressions of the Feet Obtained?

Custom cast impressions are required to make a pair of orthotics. They are obtained in the foot doctor's office with plaster-of-Paris casting material. The casts are easily removed once hardened. Some offices have computers that scan the feet for the impressions. Regardless of the technique, it's important to obtain impressions of each foot in the supported position. This ensures that the feet are maintained in the supported position while wearing the orthotics.

Allow me to expand on one of my pet peeves. The concept of getting impressions of the feet while standing has never made any sense to me. When standing and bearing all the body weight, the feet are in the collapsed position. If orthotics are made from these impressions, the resulting orthotics will only keep the feet in the same collapsed position! It doesn't matter if you are standing on a pressure plate, in a foam box, or in a puddle of plaster-of-Paris—the feet are collapsed!

I can't tell you how many patients come into the office wearing orthotics made this way. They complain that the orthotics do not help. I specifically want to know if the impressions of their feet were made when they were sitting or standing. As soon as the patient starts to say, "I was standing on . . . blah blah blah . . . this or that," I already know the orthotics are not going to provide support. When I watch the patient stand on the orthotics in the office, I can plainly see the feet are still collapsed—while they are standing on the orthotics!

In these situations, the last thing I want to do is to make another pair of useless, custom-made orthotics. However, I want to find out whether or not orthotics made with the feet in the supported position will work better than those made with the feet in the collapsed position. This is particularly true for non-diabetes-related conditions like plantar fasciitis or heel pain. As it turns out, we have a way of determining whether or not custom orthotics would be effective, even before we make them. This is especially helpful for patients who have never had orthotics.

How Do I Know if Custom Orthotics Will Work before I Order Them?

Fabricating a pair of quality custom orthotics takes a lot of time and energy. For patients with proper sensation and no neuropathy, we want to know if the pain will be eliminated with proper support and whether or not making orthotics would be worthwhile. I tell patients that I don't want to simply make a pair of custom orthotics, throw them in the shoes, and say, "Gee, I really hope these will work well for you. Good luck!" Instead, I want to know if the custom orthotics made in the supported manner will help before I make them. I do so by applying Dr. Ralph Dye's low-Dye strapping.

The low-Dye strapping is a taping technique that acts like a pair of custom orthotics. The patient leaves the strapping on the foot for five days. Patients are encouraged to be as active as possible during this testing period. They use a plastic bag while bathing or showering to keep it dry. By the end of the fifth day, the patient will know whether or not keeping the feet in the supported position feels better. If so, we know that custom orthotics fabricated in the supported position will be helpful.

The low-Dye strapping is for non-neuropathic patients who have foot pain for one reason or another. Quite frankly, when I tell patients that I am going to tape their foot, many of them look at me in disbelief. They wonder how taping their foot could do much of anything. But their faces light up as they get up from the treatment chair and put that strapped foot onto the floor because they feel better almost immediately because of the support.

It does not make sense to apply a low-Dye strapping to a neuropathic patient. These patients don't have pain. We make custom orthotics for neuropathic patients to accommodate deformities to help heal or prevent ulcers.

Custom-Made Shoes

Custom-made shoes are made from cast impressions of the feet. They are often made with leather uppers and rubber soles but can be assembled from a variety of materials. They are often larger than regular shoes because they must accommodate the deformed foot and the custom orthotics. The gold standard to prevent ulcers, amputations, and other significant complications is to put a neuropathic diabetic with poor circulation on custom orthotics in custom-made shoes.

Chapter 8

FOOT SURGERY AND DIABETES

Many doctors have told their diabetic patients that they should never have foot surgery. They fear that the foot is guaranteed to get infected or develop gangrene. The reality is that foot surgery can be the most appropriate treatment for many situations. Of course, there are special considerations involved in foot surgery on a diabetic, but these are obvious to most foot doctors. A good foot doctor will ensure proper glucose control and adequate circulation. Every situation is unique, and other considerations are often necessary.

Foot surgery is safely performed even in cases of advanced peripheral neuropathy. Just because a person has neuropathy does not mean they have poor circulation. And just because a person has poor circulation does not mean they have neuropathy.

Poor circulation is due to reduced blood flow in the arteries. Peripheral neuropathy is due to the malfunction of the nerves going to the feet. A patient may have one, the other, or both. Many people come into the office saying that they know they have poor circulation because of the funny feelings they get in their legs and feet. This may be peripheral neuropathy, but it does not necessarily indicate poor circulation.

With peripheral neuropathy, patients may feel like they have poor circulation. But some of the numbest people with the worst peripheral neuropathy can have the best circulation. A good foot doctor will evaluate the circulation to the feet in order to determine if the patient is a good candidate for surgery or not. Many patients with diabetic peripheral neuropathy are excellent surgical candidates. Elective surgical procedures are done on diabetic patients every day. Some are simple and straightforward, while others are complex. Many are performed to eliminate or prevent ulcers.

Common Conditions and Foot Surgery

Metatarsalgia

Metatarsalgia is when the bones beneath the ball of the foot become bruised. These bones are called the metatarsals, and there's one metatarsal bone behind each of the five toes. The five metatarsal bones make up the ball of the foot.

Normally, the thick fat pad beneath the five bones cushions the bottom of the foot. It acts as a protective pillow between the metatarsals and the shoe or floor. When this fat pad thins over the years, it's called *atrophy of the plantar fat pad*. The bones become bruised as they become more prominent with the loss of cushion. This is very painful with normal sensation.

Sometimes, patients think this condition is due to old age. It's not. I tell my patients it's due to high mileage! It's like when your tire tread thins out after you've driven many miles. So, too, the fat pad thins out after years of walking.

As the fat pad deteriorates, the protective cushion is reduced, and the bones become more prominent. In some cases, the bones literally protrude out from the bottom of the foot and are covered only by skin. At this point, patients are basically walking on the bones. This creates tremendous pressure on the skin, which leads to abundant amounts of callus forming on the bottom of the ball of the foot.

Plantarflexed Metatarsal Deformity

The plantarflexed metatarsal deformity is a condition in which one of the metatarsals is lower than the rest. The skin beneath that one prominent bone is subjected to significantly increased pressure leading to corn, callus, or ulcer formation.

Conservative treatment reduces the plantar pressure by debriding the lesions, padding, and off-loading the prominent bone. Surgery is considered when conservative treatments fail to reduce lesions or alleviate pain.

The surgery involves reducing the bony prominence by either lifting up the bone or shaving down the bottom of the bone. Various surgical procedures are performed to redistribute the pressure more evenly beneath the entire ball of the foot.

Metatarsalgia due to atrophy of the plantar fat pad with a plantarflexed metatarsal deformity is very common and very painful. Many patients go to the foot doctor with this condition as their chief complaint. Some only have pain beneath the ball of their foot, but most have lesions that need to be addressed. This condition is also common with rheumatoid arthritis.

Hammertoe

A hammertoe is the bending of any of the smaller toes that leads to the prominence of bone. The classic hammertoe is when there's a prominent knuckle on top of the toe, but sometimes, the bone protrudes to the left or to the right. Occasionally, an upside-down hammertoe has the bone protruding downward toward the ground. Some hammertoes are bent in multiple directions, with multiple lesions present on different sides of the same toe.

Conservative treatment includes debriding the lesions, padding, and altering the shoes to accommodate the bony prominence.

Hammertoe surgery involves removing a piece of bone from the largest of the three toe bones while straightening the toe. This reduces or eliminates the corn, callus, or ulcer. Often, the tendon that functions to elevate the toe off the ground is also lengthened or altered to reduce the upward pull on the toe. Pins are temporarily placed to hold the toe in the corrected position. Some pins stay in the toe forever. Hammertoe surgery does not involve "breaking the toe."

Bone Spurs

A bone spur, called an *exostosis*, is additional bone that grows above and beyond the normal surface of a bone. Some people call these calcium deposits. Bone spurs can form on any bone in the body. The most well-known bone spur is on the bottom of the heel—a heel spur.

Bone spurs exert increased pressure on the skin. Conservative care includes debriding lesions, padding the area, and altering the shoes. Surgery involves reducing the bony prominence when conservative care fails to manage the problem.

Foot surgeries resemble wood-working class, but with sterile tools. Bony prominences are reduced and smoothed using a variety of saws, rotary burrs, pins, wires, and screws.

Bunions

A bunion is the deformity associated with protrusion of bone behind the big toe, with the big toe often leaning into the second toe. Sometimes, the big toe leans over so much that it sits under the second toe. The prominent bump behind the big toe is from the inward tilt of the first metatarsal bone. This misalignment eventually leads to arthritis of the big toe joint. Various surgical procedures are available to reduce the size of the bump, straighten the toe, and realign the big toe joint.

Bunionettes

A bunionette, also known as a tailor's bunion, is the deformity associated with a protruding bone behind the little toe. It's the mirror opposite of a bunion. The bump behind the little toe is the fifth metatarsal that protrudes outward, while the little toe leans into the fourth toe. Various surgical procedures can reduce the bump, straighten the little toe, and realign the fifth toe joint.

Foot doctors take X-rays of the foot to evaluate the level of deformity and joint misalignment. Knowing the degree of arthritis also helps determine the most appropriate surgical procedure.

Ulcers

Ulcers are defects in the skin usually caused by pressure with bony deformity and poor circulation. They are the enemy of the diabetic foot. There are other types of ulcers, but our focus is on the diabetic foot ulcer, DFU. Neuropathy, pressure, and poor circulation contribute to ulcer formation, persistence, and failure to heal.

People without neuropathy can feel the pain associated with increased pressure on the skin, which results in some sort of response to eliminate the cause. At the very least, the patient will realize that something's wrong and will look at their foot. Pain is a good thing because it helps avoid injury and damage.

However, if you have neuropathy, the pressure persists because you can't feel the pain. Eventually, the integrity of your skin will be compromised, and an ulcer forms. The situation worsens because if you can't feel it, the ulcer grows larger and then becomes infected. This is why you must look at your feet every day if you have neuropathy. Many problems can be discovered and circumvented simply by looking at your feet.

Look inside your shoes too. All kinds of debris end up in shoes. A small pebble can cause havoc by rolling around in the shoe all day, which you won't feel if you have neuropathy. Debris in your shoes can tear open the skin, and if you don't look inside your shoes, you'll have no idea that it's happening.

Never walk barefooted. Even wearing a simple house shoe will protect the bottom of your feet from debris.

Never walk barefooted. Even wearing a simple house shoe will protect the bottom of your feet from debris.

Ulcer Classifications

Diabetic foot ulcers are complex and often require care from multiple specialists. Various classification schemes have been created to describe ulcers.

Wagner Classification System

Dr. F.W. Wagner created one of the first classification systems to describe diabetic foot ulcers. The six grades, from 0 to 5, describe the depth of the ulcer, the involvement of bone, and the level of gangrene.[7]

- Grade 0: healed ulcer on a high-risk foot
- Grade 1: ulcer involving a defect in the skin, but not beneath the skin
- Grade 2: ulcer involving the skin, and ligaments or muscle, but no bone
- Grade 3: ulcer to bone with bone infection
- Grade 4: ulcer with gangrene of the forefoot
- Grade 5: ulcer with gangrene of the entire foot

The Wagner system had been used for years but eventually became too simplistic as the understanding of ulcers evolved over time.

---

[7] Wagner, F.W. Jr., "The Diabetic Foot," *Orthopedics* 1987; 10:163–72

The University of Texas Wound Classification System of Diabetic Foot Ulcers

This system has largely replaced the Wagner system.[8] The twelve grades of this system are more descriptive by including the depth of the ulcer, the presence of infection, and the degree of circulation.

- Grade IA: non-infected, non-ischemic superficial ulceration (non-ischemic is a double negative as it means no poor circulation, which means good circulation is present)
- Grade IB: infected, non-ischemic superficial ulceration
- Grade IC: ischemic, non-infected superficial ulceration (ischemic means poor circulation)
- Grade ID: ischemic and infected superficial ulceration
- Grade IIA: non-infected, non-ischemic ulcer that penetrates to capsule or tendon
- Grade IIB: infected, non-ischemic ulcer that penetrates to capsule or tendon
- Grade IIC: ischemic, non-infected ulcer that penetrates to capsule or tendon
- Grade IID: ischemic and infected ulcer that penetrates to capsule or tendon
- Grade IIIA: non-infected, non-ischemic ulcer that penetrates to bone or joint
- Grade IIIB: infected, non-ischemic ulcer that penetrates to bone or joint

---

[8] Lavery, L.A.; Armstrong ,D.G.; Harkless, L.B., "Classification of Diabetic Foot Wounds," *Journal of Foot and Ankle Surgery* 35, (1996), 528–31.

- Grade IIIC: ischemic, non-infected ulcer that penetrates to bone or joint
- Grade IIID: ischemic and infected ulcer that penetrates to bone or joint

SINBAD Classification System[9]

The SINBAD classification system assigns points for various characteristics of the ulcer. The prognosis worsens with a higher score. SINBAD is an acronym for:

- **S**ite: location of the ulcer (0 points if located on the forefoot, awarded 1 point if located on the hindfoot)
- **I**schemia: intact or poor circulation (0 points for palpable pulses, awarded 1 point for non-palpable pulses)
- **N**europathy: protective sensation intact or lost (0 points if intact, awarded 1 point if lost)
- **B**acterial Infection: ulcer infection absent or present (0 points if absent, awarded 1 point if infected)
- **A**rea: ulcer measurement (0 points if less than 1 square cm, awarded 1 point if larger than 1 square cm)
- **D**epth: ulcer depth (0 points if ulcer is confined to skin and subcutaneous tissues, awarded 1 point if depth reaches muscle, tendon, or deeper)

Other classification systems exist, and even more are being developed. No single classification system can describe every ulcer, but these systems are used to communicate between

---

[9] Ince, Paul, et al. "Use of the SINBAD Classification System and Score in Comparing Outcome of Foot Ulcer Management on Three Continents," *Diabetes Care*, Volume 31, May 1, 2008, 964–967.

healthcare providers and monitor ulcers as they heal or worsen over time.

Why Don't Ulcers Heal?

Why does the skin break down when exposed to pressure? Why does the body become unable to heal the ulcer? Why do diabetics take longer to heal than non-diabetics? There are no simple answers, but we do know that the ability of your body to repair itself is reduced with long-standing diabetes.

Many factors contribute to the reduced ability to heal diabetic wounds. Pressure, neuropathy, altered collagen synthesis, reduced immune system function, and reduced blood flow all play a part. The trifecta of diabetes—neuropathy, pressure, and poor circulation—cause many ulcers that become difficult to heal.

Collagen is a protein and is the primary connective tissue that makes up most of the body, including the skin. The body uses collagen to heal itself. It's believed that the synthesis of this protein becomes altered and abnormal with long-standing diabetes. This is the primary reason why the body loses the ability to repair itself.

The trifecta of diabetes—neuropathy, pressure, and poor circulation—cause many ulcers that become difficult to heal.

Over time, diabetics develop thicker, rubbery, less-pliable skin. The turgor is gone, and the skin becomes less elastic and more rigid. This condition is known as *diabetic dermopathy*. Skin in this state is more susceptible to damage and ulceration and has a reduced ability to heal.

Poor circulation contributes to poor healing because the required growth factors necessary for healing simply can't get to the site of injury. Immune system suppression also diminishes the body's ability to heal by preventing messenger proteins from being sent out. These proteins would normally tell the body that a repair is necessary.

The delay in response to injury and the reduced ability to heal a wound allows the damage to worsen with time. It also allows bacteria to enter the area, which leads to infection. Diabetics take longer to heal because the healing process becomes abnormal.

Pressure on the skin is the initial factor that leads to an ulcer. Pressure creates a relatively small injury that doesn't properly heal. Ongoing pressure leads to cumulative injuries and ultimately to the loss of integrity.

Wound Care

Wound care is the mainstay of ulcer treatment. It involves removing tissues that interfere with healing, eliminating infection, and creating an environment conducive to healing the wound. *Debridement* is the physical act of removing tissues that interfere with healing. Topical or oral antibiotics eliminate infection, while dressings help provide an optimal wound healing environment. Circulation to the area may be improved with medication or surgery.

There's a common myth regarding wound healing that says to leave the wound open to the air, so it can dry out and form a scab. This is an "old wives' tale" because it's not true. Dry wounds take longer to heal. Wounds that are kept covered and moist heal quicker than dry wounds.

Advanced Treatments for Ulcers

Advanced treatments are employed when local care fails to heal the ulcer. This can include topical medications that provide growth factors, various wound dressings that optimize the wound environment, and skin substitutes that replace defects in the skin.

A wound vacuum, or *wound vac*, is a medical-grade vacuum similar to the one you have at home. They're usually reserved for large, deep defects that are difficult to heal. Wound vacs apply a constant negative sucking pressure that reduces swelling and provides a better wound healing environment.

Hyperbaric oxygen therapy (HBOT) exposes the patient and the wound to elevated levels of oxygen. HBOT creates an environment with about two-and-a-half times the normal level of oxygen. In this treatment, the entire person is placed in a see-through glass chamber for thirty minutes to two hours several times per week. The elevated oxygen level helps wounds heal.

The historical gold standard of wound care was to place the patient into a total contact cast (TCC). These casts were put on to accommodate the specific contours and deformities of the foot. Are you surprised to learn that not all casts are for broken bones? The next cast you see may be for a diabetic ulcer. TCC greatly reduces plantar pressures and is applied for Charcot foot and difficult to heal plantar ulcers.

An entire medical community is devoted to wound care, which has led to the creation of many wound care centers. Foot doctors, vascular surgeons, and wound care physicians work as a team to treat difficult-to-heal ulcers at these centers.

Charcot Foot

Charcot foot, named for Dr. Jean-Martin Charcot (1825–1893), who first described this condition, is a very destructive process that occurs only when neuropathy is present. In this condition, the bones and joints in the middle of the foot break into many pieces, causing an irreversible collapse of the arch. Often, large bony prominences protrude downward toward the ground. The dramatic, increased pressure beneath these prominent bones leads to the loss of skin integrity and ulceration. The ulcers are typically large and difficult to heal. Charcot foot sometimes attacks the ankle instead of the midfoot.

Symptoms Of Charcot Foot

The destructive nature of Charcot foot leads to an inflammatory response by the body. The typical characteristics of a Charcot flair include significant swelling, redness, and warmth of the newly deformed foot.

Causes Of Charcot Foot

Charcot foot only occurs when neuropathy is present, which happens with diseases other than diabetes. However, the overwhelming majority of neuropathy is from diabetes. There are two theories that help explain the cause of Charcot foot:

1. The "Neurotraumatic" theory suggests that unperceived repetitive trauma or injury to the numb foot causes ongoing microfractures. The microfractures progress to large fractures and then deformity.
2. The "Neurovascular" theory suggests that the increased vascular flow to the bones washes away a portion of the bone density. The thinner bones weaken and become more susceptible to fracture and collapse.

You may recall that nerves normally maintain the muscles around the arteries in a partially contracted state. Neuropathy allows the muscles around the arteries to relax, dilating the arteries. This creates a huge increase in blood flow to the bones. This increased blood flow is thought to wash away some of the bone stock, leading to fracture and collapse.

Most cases of Charcot foot happen without a specific injury or trauma. Most sufferers don't recall tripping, falling, or hitting their foot against any furniture. Yet, a specific injury can precipitate the onset of Charcot foot.

Treatment of Charcot Foot

The bony destruction seen in Charcot foot progresses quickly. Treatment needs to be initiated immediately to curtail the magnitude of collapse and deformity. However, treatment cannot begin until the correct diagnosis is made. Charcot foot is often misdiagnosed as gout, infection, arthritis, or a sprained foot, which can all cause a warm, red, swollen foot. The possibility of Charcot foot must be considered by the patient and the doctor when these symptoms are present. X-rays usually confirm the diagnosis by demonstrating the typical fracture pattern across the midfoot.

Once the diagnosis is made, limiting the extent of the destruction is the goal of treatment. The *acute* phase includes swelling, redness, and warmth, with rapid, progressive bone and joint destruction. Immediately, patients cease bearing weight on that foot, which is immobilized in a boot or cast to curtail the destructive process. Patients stay off the affected foot until the acute phase subsides, usually several days to several weeks.

Some receive additional medicine that helps slow down the bony destruction. One of the more commonly used drugs comes in the form of a nasal spray. Your doctor may prescribe such a spray to curtail the bony collapse in your foot.

The *subacute* phase of Charcot foot is achieved when the foot calms down. The swelling reduces, the redness and warmth fade, and the bony destruction has ceased. The foot is deformed but calm.

The *chronic* phase of Charcot foot is when all the fracture fragments coalesce into a big blob of bone in the middle of the foot. The foot is irreversibly deformed but stable. The initial inflammation and redness are long gone. Treatment is now geared toward returning the patient to a safe, weight-bearing status while preventing ulceration. Most require custom inserts and custom shoes to accommodate the deformity and offload the pressure to prominent bones. Surgery may now be considered to reduce bony prominences, particularly on the bottom of the midfoot. Some have Charcot reconstruction to try to restore a more natural contour, knowing that achieving a normal arch is almost impossible.

Charcot foot is a complex condition that requires ongoing management for the rest of the person's life. The primary goal is to return the patient to full weight-bearing status while avoiding ulcers.

A FINAL WORD

I hope this book has given you a better understanding of the diabetic foot and that the information has made you feel less afraid and more informed. My goal is to motivate you to take better care of your diabetes and your feet. Paying attention to your feet truly helps prevent all kinds of problems. I wish you good health and happy feet!

Appendix A

QUESTIONS FOR YOUR DOCTOR

Questions to Ask at Every Visit

How does the skin on my feet look to you today?

How is my circulation?

Do I have neuropathy?

Is there anything between my toes or on the bottom of my feet?

How do my toenails look?

How are my shoes?

Do I have the "trifecta of diabetes" (deformity, neuropathy, and poor circulation)?

For additional information, visit the American Diabetes Association website at www.diabetes.org.

ABOUT THE AUTHOR

Dr. Randy Aaranson was born and raised in Philadelphia, Pennsylvania. He moved to Saint Louis, Missouri, in 1989 and began practicing podiatry after residency in 1991. He's married to his wife, Rochelle, and they have three children—Jeremy, Sydney, and Ethan—none of whom like science or medicine! Dr. Aaranson plays ice hockey, golf, and poker. He loves to be near the ocean and is an accomplished cook.

www.ingramcontent.com/pod-product-compliance
Lightning Source LLC
Chambersburg PA
CBHW050505120526
44589CB00047B/2361